MW00472739

Pediatric Ethics

PEDIATRIC ETHICS

Protecting the Interests of Children

Alan R. Fleischman, M.D.

OXFORD
UNIVERSITY PRESS

OXFORD
UNIVERSITY PRESS

Oxford University Press is a department of the University of Oxford. It furthers
the University's objective of excellence in research, scholarship, and education
by publishing worldwide.Oxford is a registered trade mark of Oxford University
Press in the UK and certain other countries.

Published in the United States of America by Oxford University Press
198 Madison Avenue, New York, NY 10016, United States of America.

© Oxford University Press 2016

All rights reserved. No part of this publication may be reproduced, stored in
a retrieval system, or transmitted, in any form or by any means, without the
prior permission in writing of Oxford University Press, or as expressly permitted
by law, by license, or under terms agreed with the appropriate reproduction
rights organization. Inquiries concerning reproduction outside the scope of the
above should be sent to the Rights Department, Oxford University Press, at the
address above.

You must not circulate this work in any other form
and you must impose this same condition on any acquirer.

Names: Fleischman, Alan R., author.
Title: Pediatric ethics : protecting the interests of children / Alan R. Fleischman.
Description: New York, NY : Oxford University Press, [2016] | Includes
bibliographical references and index.
Identifiers: LCCN 2015049222 | ISBN 9780199354474 (pbk. : alk. paper)
Subjects: | MESH: Pediatrics—ethics | Bioethical Issues | Child
Health—ethics | Patient Rights—ethics | United States
Classification: LCC RJ47.8 | NLM WS 21 | DDC 174.2/9892—dc23 LC record available at
http://lccn.loc.gov/2015049222

9 8 7 6 5 4 3 2 1

Printed by Webcom, Inc., Canada

CONTENTS

ACKNOWLEDGMENT

I am grateful to countless patients and their families who have allowed me into their lives during times of serious illness and great distress. My personal values and professional skills were meaningfully affected by these interactions.

This book is dedicated to those families, to my colleagues and students who have taught me so much, and to my own family, without whose love and support nothing is possible.

CHAPTER 1

Children Are Special

Hard Questions, Hard Choices

In the 21st century, children's lives are being saved because of remarkable advances in biomedical research and clinical care. Assisted reproduction, prenatal and fetal genetic testing, advances in neonatal intensive care, sophisticated pediatric critical care, increasing use of solid organ and bone marrow transplantation, and a burgeoning number of drugs and surgical interventions for "enhancement," are all available to potentially enrich the lives of children. These treatments and technologies bring not only the promise of longer and better lives, but also the possibility of creating extraordinary burdens and a diminished quality of life for children. How can we best use these modern treatments and technologies in a thoughtful and appropriate manner that assures the interests of children? As parents and clinicians caring for critically and chronically ill children, we are faced with many hard choices that will dramatically affect these children, their families, and the broader society. The goal of this book is to explore many complex medical issues that generate hard questions about healthcare decision-making for children, and to assist clinicians and parents to make wise choices consistent with the best interests of each individual child.

I am a pediatrician and a neonatologist (newborn specialist) who has been committed to helping children and advocating for their interests for over 50 years. I am a father and a grandfather, but long before I had a child I knew that children needed loving families and deserved very special attention in order to develop and optimize their potential.

I never met a newborn I didn't like. I can't say that about all children and certainly not about all their parents. But all children are special; they are inherently vulnerable and require nurturance and protection. Children bring joy and happiness to families. Children also demand a great deal and can create great challenges for parents. They do not ask to be brought into the world and they do not choose their families or siblings. We should not blame them for arriving among us and we should not be surprised if they are different from what we expected.

Every baby is different and each family has different hopes and expectations for their child. Ask any baby-nurse or parent and they will confirm that newborns have unique personalities from the moment of birth. Each child responds differently, has different needs and desires, and attaches to his or her caregivers in a distinctive way. Interacting with young children and unraveling the keys to their personalities is a great mystery and one of the great joys of my life. Parents bring different strengths and capacities to the process of relating to a new baby or a young child and sometimes ask more of their young infants than the child can deliver. Children are easy to love if we merely open ourselves to their world and ask little in return, but children can be a disappointment to their parents if they do not fulfill their parents' inappropriate expectations.

So why do people have children? Fifty percent of pregnancies are unplanned. That is not to say that half the children who are born are unwanted. Although planning a pregnancy and wishing to have a child should ensure that a child is desired, that, too, is not always the case. People have children for all kinds of reasons. We would hope that parents have children in order to create a new person whose needs and welfare are primary and for whom they wish to provide a loving and nurturing environment. Yet, children are often created to fulfill parents' needs and desires, the need to be loved, to be supported, to be cared for in old age, and the desire to perpetuate a genetic lineage or to create an enhanced self in one's own image.

As adults, we hope that our children will grow up to share our values and admire our behaviors; yet as children, we often criticize our parents' values and behaviors. We also want to be different from our parents in childrearing practices, but our parents are the closest role models we have when we are faced with parenthood. Our parents' words that we disliked as a child can often be heard emanating from our mouths, and parental behaviors we disliked are too frequently imitated. There is little formal education provided to most of us on how to be a good parent, and even less preparation for how to be a good parent to a child who is sick.

It is always sad when children are sick and unable to demonstrate the natural vitality and joy that is so much a part of being a child. Parents, family members, pediatricians, and other health professionals are often emotionally unprepared when faced with caring for a sick child. And they are often devastated by the possibility that a child may die or suffer irreversible damage that results in profound limitations on their future potential. Parents and clinicians face many hard questions about what is the right health care decision for a sick child. Parents ask themselves, "What would a good parent do in this situation?" Clinicians ask, "How can I fulfill my obligations to my patient and to his or her family?" And both ask, "What is best for the child?"

As I interacted with a large number of families of critically ill children, I was struck that virtually all wanted what was best for their child but there was wide variation in the values that were expressed. Some families were willing to allow their child to die by withholding or withdrawing medical treatments when prognosis was poor, others were steadfast about continuing treatments when there was any possible hope for continued survival regardless of future quality of life, and still others were unable to make decisions in these situations. Personal values were sometimes based on ethnic or religious background, but more often values were based on life experiences, cultural norms, economic status, and perceptions of what it meant to be a "good" parent. Often a family would ask me, "What would you do if this were your child?" I recognized that this question was another way of saying: "What do you think is the best choice for my child?" I never answered the question about what I would do if it were my child, but I was always willing to make recommendations about what I thought was best for their child based on my best medical advice and what I heard from them about their views and values. I feared that if I told them what I would do if it were my child, they would be coerced into accepting that choice even if they disagreed; and if they did disagree, they would be unable to tell me for fear that I would think less of them for the choice they preferred.

I also learned that doctors have a wide range of values, and differing views on their obligations to impose those values on their patients. Some physicians are reluctant to ever withhold or withdraw treatments from patients, believing that a fundamental goal of medicine is to save lives, almost at any cost in dollars or human suffering. Other doctors do not value those who are different or disabled and are reluctant to provide aggressive treatment to such patients. Some doctors are strongly motivated by their own religious views and believe they are obligated to practice medicine based on those views, even if their patients do not share them. And many doctors, in the age of evidence-based medicine, have great difficulty providing different treatment plans for patients with similar medical conditions, when patients or families have different views about what is best.

Early in my career, I recognized that much of my work involved making recommendations about treatment decisions for critically and chronically ill children in the face of great uncertainty about the ultimate benefits and burdens of these interventions. I observed distraught and overwhelmed parents trusting physicians to make the right decisions for their children. I was taught by senior physicians who were reluctant to admit to parents that their treatment recommendations were not merely medical choices based on the best medical evidence but, rather, value choices based in personal views of what constitutes a life worth living. During these formative years in my career, I pondered several critical questions: When is it right to stop treatment for a critically ill child? Who should decide when to withhold or withdraw life-sustaining treatments? Should doctors protect families from having to make difficult and painful healthcare decisions for their children? Was it the obligation of a physician to save a child's life regardless of the future quality of that life? Did the fact that some children had been saved and went on to flourish as a result of a specific treatment make it mandatory that all children in similar medical circumstances be provided that care? Or should children with similar medical conditions be treated differently based on family values and preferences? These were just a few of the questions that seemed part of my daily practice and drew me to the field of ethics in order to explore reasonable answers.

My early attempts to find answers to these questions brought me to collaborate with and learn from scholars at The Hastings Center, the first bioethics center in the United States, and to assist in the creation of the infant bioethics program at Montefiore Medical Center and the Albert Einstein College of Medicine in the Bronx, New York. As the director of the neonatal program, I was responsible for the care of thousands of children each year. I was fortunate to find colleagues in philosophy and law as well as thoughtful clinicians in medicine, nursing, and social work who helped me to find tentative answers to my questions and to learn how to do ethical analyses of complex issues. Because of my personal and academic interest in exploring these issues, I was appointed as a founding member of the New York State Governor's Task Force on Life and the Law, the state bioethics commission, that wrote comprehensive reports and successfully catalyzed state legislation and regulation on end-of-life decision-making, brain death, assisted reproductive technologies, genetic testing, surrogate parenting, organ donation, and many other critical issues at the intersection of medicine, science, law, and ethics. As a member of the American Academy of Pediatrics Bioethics Committee for six years, I helped deal with the "Baby Doe" crisis created by federal regulations that threatened to separate parents from input on decisions for their critically ill and dying infants. All these experiences brought me in contact with a small group of pediatricians, nurses, mental health professionals, philosophers and lawyers who shared similar interests and concerns, and we, together, were responsible for the creation of the field of pediatric ethics.

PEDIATRIC ETHICS

Pediatric ethics is a part of the larger field of bioethics. Bioethics, focused on healthcare delivery and research involving human subjects, is the study of moral conduct and the rational process for determining the best course of action in the face of conflicting choices. Bioethics is about resolving conflicts of values and conflicts of obligations and duties. Through careful and thoughtful analysis, bioethics should help each of us to justify our decisions when making difficult health-related choices for ourselves or others. Since truly difficult ethical choices are not those between good and evil, but between one good and another good, bioethics provides guidance to examine conflicts and prioritize choices among reasonable options. Making the best choice is not just a matter of opinion, some choices are better than others, more informed, more respectful of the interests of the person for whom the decision is being made, more consistent with the values of that person and other involved stakeholders, and more aware of the breadth of the available choices.

Pediatric ethics applies the field of bioethics to children; those who are not yet born and those who are in our midst. All decisions for children, at least those children who are young and unable to decide for themselves, are surrogate decisions made by others, usually parents. Young children are particularly vulnerable, their wishes have never been expressed and their views and values cannot be elicited. They are thus subject to the values of others and may suffer the long-term consequences of decisions in which they did not participate. Pediatric ethics explores how to make the best choices for children. It seeks to define parental and clinician obligations to children and most importantly, it attempts to protect the interests of children.

When considering complex health-related decisions, bioethics describes several ways in which to ethically ground such judgments. Ethical choices can be grounded and justified through examination of principles, oaths, or consequences. Principles are rules that can be invoked to govern behavior. Oaths are contracts or promises made in the past that govern present behavior. Consequences are the use of a careful analysis of likely benefits and likely burdens or harms of each possible choice to make the decision that produces the most benefit and the least harm.

Principles

Principles are rules, and ethical choices are those decisions consistent with agreed upon principles. At times principles may come in conflict and the need arises to prioritize one principle over another. In bioethics, three principles have emerged over the past 40 years that have been extraordinarily well accepted and seemingly helpful in grounding ethical judgments: respect for autonomy, beneficence, and justice. Respect for autonomy asserts that each person who has the capacity to decide has the right to make healthcare decisions for him- or herself based on their own values and views of what is best. Persons with autonomy may even refuse life-sustaining treatments that others deem to be in their interests. This principle creates two correlative duties on the part of health professionals. First, to offer all treatments reasonably thought to be in the patient's interest; and second, not to impose a procedure or treatment on a patient without their informed permission. The principle of respect for autonomy invokes a negative right, the right to refuse offered treatments. This principle does not provide for the positive right of a patient or family to demand a treatment that is not medically indicated and not offered.

Respect for autonomy as a principle has limited applicability in pediatric ethics because young children do not have the capacity to make decisions for themselves. But when decisions are being contemplated for older children and adolescents, the concept of evolving autonomy requires decision-makers to at least consider the views and values of the patient. Some believe that the principle of respect for autonomy is applicable when a parent is making a health-related decision for their child. But respect for autonomy allows the capacitated decision-maker to refuse any medical treatment. Should there be any limits to parental discretion in refusing treatments for their children that are different from refusing treatments for themselves? And should a parent's request for treatment be respected when clinicians feel that such treatment is not in the interests of the patient?

The second principle, beneficence, asserts that in relationships with another person our recommendations and decisions should maximize benefits and minimize harms to them. Our own conflicting and competing interests should be excluded, focusing primarily on the interests of the person for whom we are deciding. This principle has been seen as fundamental to the obligation of parents when considering health-related decisions for their children. Beneficence is also at the core of the duty of clinicians to make recommendations to their patients that maximize the patient's interests. It is the basis of the trust a patient generally feels when being treated by a health professional, even if there is no prior relationship between the two. Patients and parents believe that health professionals are motivated by the principle of beneficence and accept that their doctor or nurse will recommend procedures or treatments that are in their interests, maximizing benefits and minimizing harms as best possible.

Beneficence is a powerfully important principle in pediatric ethics; it creates duties and expectations not only on the part of health professionals to maximize benefits for children but also on the part of parents. It is clear that the principle of beneficence may come in conflict with the principle of respect for autonomy when parents are making health-related decisions for their children. When should a clinician's view of what constitutes maximizing the benefits for a child override the decision of a parent? Even if we prioritize the principle of beneficence over respect for autonomy, that does not solve the problem. Since clinicians and parents may have differing views of what constitutes maximizing the interests of an individual child, it is easy to see how the application of the principle of beneficence could result in conflicting views of what is best.

In attempting to sort out these conflicts, many invoke the concept of "the best interest of the child," as the standard that should be utilized in making beneficence-based judgments. At first glance, the best-interest standard makes sense, since everyone might agree that we ought to attempt to enhance a child's interest when making decisions for him or her. But, the concept of best interest is a very subjective and individualistic assessment that may not resolve the conflict. Although not perfect, the concept of best interest can be very useful in focusing the discussion on what's at stake for the child from the perspective of the child. While accepting that the concept of best interest is subjective, this concept can be helpful to remind decision-makers that the child should be the primary focus of decision-making. Inevitably, there will be conflicts between parents and between parents and clinicians when there are differing views of what is in the best interest of a child, and there will need to be resolution of these conflicts. Pediatric ethics may be helpful in these situations.

The third principle, justice, incorporates fairness into choices that affect others. When dividing a cake, some might argue that providing an equal share to each person is fair and just. But in the face of unequal need such as in the case of a person who is sick or a community that is poor, fairness might require an equitable rather than an equal distribution of resources, based on need. The principle of justice is often invoked in pediatric ethics in discussions of social responsibility, access to care, allocation of organs, and the availability of high-quality treatment for poor children. The principle of justice also plays an important role in the analysis of the appropriate methods to encourage participation in research, ensuring that those who will be exposed to the risks of research are a part of the population that will be able to derive benefit from the findings of the research.

Oaths

Oaths are promises made in the past that govern present behavior. Virtually every physician in the United States upon graduation from medical school takes an oath promising to uphold the ethical standards of the profession including: competence, confidentiality, altruism, truth telling, and so forth. Oaths can be important in motivating behavior, but the mandated action comes from a promise made in the past that may or may not be sufficiently specific or relevant to the present circumstances.

Consequences

Assessing consequences includes a careful analysis of likely benefits and likely burdens or harms of each possible choice in order to make the decision that produces the most benefit and the least harm. This approach is done contemporaneously and includes the obligation not to trivialize negative consequences or overestimate likely benefits. Although doing a good consequentialist analysis is difficult, it is used on a daily basis by clinicians in making all kinds of recommendations to patients about procedures and treatments. Health professionals are comfortable with consequentialist analysis and use this approach frequently even when there are no evident value conflicts.

In the chapters ahead, we will use principles, promises, and analysis of consequences to assist in examining many issues in pediatric ethics. The goal will be to define the important ethical questions in each area and to provide a thorough analysis utilizing whatever tools seem best. Although there will sometimes be proposed answers to the questions, at other times answers will not be clear and we will be left with options and choices that the reader will need to assess to determine what course is best.

Historically, at the beginning of the United States, parents were seen as the stewards of their children's well-being, responsible for all aspects of their care. Children were viewed as their family's property, owned particularly by the father, and able to be put to work, educated or not, and disciplined in whatever ways thought necessary. This approach to children was consistent with the federalist system that was created after the American revolution that prioritized personal and religious freedom and brought about a libertarian philosophy concerning the role of government in personal lives. In the 19th century, courts began to intervene in family matters, arguing that children were members of the society and children deserved protection from harm. Parents could discipline their children but they were not allowed to beat their children so badly as to maim them.

By the early 20th century, replicating the work of the Society for the Prevention of Cruelty to Animals, local communities passed anti-child-abuse laws, fair-child-labor-practices laws, and compulsory-education laws. These societal interventions in the lives of children made clear that not only did parents have obligations to their children but also that the greater society shared the responsibility to ensure the well-being of children. Parental decision-making authority was seen increasingly as contingent on behaving in ways that were socially responsible and not neglectful or abusive. Parents continued to exert broad authority over decisions concerning their children, but the state—through the principle of "parens patriae" or "the state as parent"—asserted state interest in protecting children and enforcing an obligation on the part of families to provide adequate safety, food, clothing, shelter, and education for their children. Some commentators balked at this diminution in parental rights and autonomy and argued that the state had no role in intervening in the private lives of families. Others argued that it was possible to maintain respect for family autonomy in general while permitting state intervention in specific cases to protect the interests of an individual child who was in danger.

By the mid-20th century in America, the moral and legal status of children was well accepted. Children were deemed to be persons. Families had moral obligations to protect the interests of their children, and the state invoked its power to enforce those obligations. Children had rights, not identical to the rights of adults, but children were considered in need of protection so that they might fulfill their inalienable right to life, liberty, and happiness when they became adults.

In 1960, despite the post-World War II economic boom in the United States, 35% of the elderly and 27% of children lived in poverty and most of these Americans had no health insurance. The vast majority of the general adult population was able to obtain health insurance through employment, whereas the retired elderly, who were most susceptible to illness, were uninsured unless they maintained that benefit as a result of prior employment. Illness in the elderly with substantial healthcare expenditures often resulted in bankruptcy, increasing the numbers in poverty. The passage of Medicare in the 1960s, universal entitlement to health insurance for those over 65, combined with Social Security, universal retirement benefits, reversed this trend and enabled the elderly to rise out of poverty and have a reasonably secure and dignified period of retirement. Because of these changes, by 2010, only 9% of the elderly lived in poverty while over 22% of children remained in poverty. Children were not afforded a similar entitlement to health insurance in the 20th century; even now the program to provide universal access to health insurance for children varies greatly among the states in both eligibility requirements and breadth of covered services. Similarly, the quality and expenditure on public education for children varies widely from state to state and among communities in an individual state.

Currently, more than one in five American children live in poverty, more than 16 million children, and over 70 million children live in families with low income as defined by an income less than two times the federal poverty level or about $44,000 for a family of four. Thus, children may be viewed as having full moral and legal status as persons in America but how much their health and future well-being are valued by our society remains unclear. Since health insurance and aid to families in poverty is determined by each state, geography has become destiny for our children by allowing wide variations among the states in provision of fundamental benefits.

Regardless of where they live, parents and families remain ultimately responsible for their children. Although the definition of family may have broadened and cultural norms changed, children are viewed today as being best served as part of a loving family within a supportive community. This implies that there will be very wide differences in values and practices of individual families within local communities and that clinicians caring for children will be faced with views, values, and preferences that may be quite different from their own. We will examine how healthcare professionals with varying values can deal with this diversity and with the potential for conflict between their own values and those of the families they care for.

This book will examine a wide spectrum of hard questions, hard choices, and value conflicts involving children, through the lens of pediatric ethics. Pediatric ethics requires an understanding of developmental biology and psychology, awareness that capacity to participate in decision-making evolves with age and experience, and respect for the important relationships that are inherent in being a parent and creating a child. Pediatric ethics is more complex and nuanced than adult ethics. Most adults make their own decisions. Most decisions for children are made by surrogates, generally their parents or legal guardians. Decisions for children tend to be collaborative among clinicians and families with patient involvement when developmentally possible. This creates the potential for value conflicts and ethical concerns among the various stakeholders. Pediatric ethics is family-centered, respecting the role of parent and family in the lives of children—roles that are fundamentally different from the role of family in the lives of adults. Pediatric ethics also recognizes special protections afforded the interests of children by society at large and the obligations of clinicians to advocate for and protect children in many ways that differ from comparable duties to adults.

The book begins by discussing the ethical issues involved in creating and giving birth to a child and moves through clinical areas related to neonatal care, general pediatric practice, end of life care, medical and surgical enhancements of children, and the care of adolescents. It also includes chapters on ethical analyses in genetic testing and screening in children, and the use of children as participants in research. I will use case examples in many of the chapters in an attempt to share the complexity and richness of real-life examples and to clarify how pediatric ethics approaches these problems.

Children begin their lives with a unique set of genetic and physical attributes that will determine only a small part of the ultimate person they will become. Their interactions with the world around them, and the decisions made for them, will have a more profound impact on their future health and well-being than their biologic makeup. My hope is that healthcare professionals and families given the authority and responsibility for making complex decisions for sick children will profit from discussions in this book and that children will be benefited by more thoughtful and wise choices made on their behalf.

CHAPTER 2
Ethical Issues in Creating a Child

Case 1

Penny Singleton, a successful 58-year-old financier presents to a fertility center for evaluation of her potential to become pregnant in order to have a baby with her new husband, John Braithwaite. Penny and John are aware that it is likely they will need donor eggs but Penny insists that she wants to carry the baby. Penny has had three children as the result of a previous marriage that ended in divorce. John, 62 years old, has never been married, has no children of his own, and would very much like to have a child with Penny. Both Penny and John are healthy and have carefully thought about the obvious fact that they will be older parents if they are successful at creating a baby.

Case 2

Pablo is a 4-year-old boy with Hodgkin's lymphoma, who has not responded to initial chemotherapy and radiation treatments and for whom the doctors recommend a hematopoietic stem cell transplant along with additional treatment. The doctors explain to Betty and Jesus Morales, Pablo's parents, that the best hope for Pablo is finding a very closely matched donor to provide the stem cells. After checking with all the public and private bone marrow donor registries and umbilical cord blood banks with no success, the doctors screen all of Pablo's very close relatives and find no match. Betty and Jesus were quite distraught until they read on the Internet about the possibility of conceiving another child of their own who would be both unaffected and a complete match for Pablo. Umbilical cord hematopoietic stem cells obtained at birth could be used to treat Pablo. Betty and Jesus were not considering having another child and they are concerned about the costs of this plan, but they are excited about the possibility that within a year they might have a new child and the needed stem cells for Pablo's treatment. They seek advice at the local reproductive endocrinology IVF program.

Case 3

Fred and Sarah Johnson, both 30 years old, have been married for three years and would like to have a baby. Sarah suffers from both Type I (juvenile) diabetes, Celiac disease, and Systemic Lupus Erythematosis that have resulted in chronic hypertension and severe kidney disease. Her doctors counsel that pregnancy could be very dangerous and will likely exacerbate her renal disease. The Johnsons decide to utilize IVF with an egg donor and a gestational surrogate to make having a baby safe and possible. Through searches on the Internet and with the help of an attorney, they identify a potential surrogate and initiate IVF with egg donation at a respected program in their city. The pregnancy goes well and the surrogate remains healthy throughout. To the surprise of the Johnsons, when the baby is born at term, the surrogate mother decides she wants to keep the baby.

Approximately four million children are born each year in the United States. With such a high number of births, you might conclude that it is pretty easy to create a baby, but at any one time, about two million couples wishing to conceive a child find that they are infertile. The accepted definition of infertility is a couple who are unable to create a pregnancy after one year of actively attempting to conceive. The prevalence of infertility has increased in the United States over the past several decades. A woman's risk of infertility rises with increasing age at first conception, chronic stress, smoking, history of pelvic infections, abnormal ovarian function, being underweight or overweight, and several medical conditions and uterine anatomic abnormalities. Men also play an important role in infertility. It is estimated that in about one-third of couples, infertility is related to abnormalities in sperm number or function.

Infertility is a very serious concern for many couples. Some commentators believe that most causes of infertility relate to social and behavioral factors such as promiscuity that increases sexually transmitted diseases, obesity, and drug use. Since these factors are a result of personal choices that are socially irresponsible, these commentators believe society should not make a significant investment in infertility treatment. Others argue that infertility is so important it must be considered a medical disorder that merits full attention from the medical community and adequate health insurance coverage for prevention, evaluation, and treatment. The prevention of infertility requires that young women beginning in childhood and continuing into adulthood receive comprehensive family planning and healthcare services. Private insurance coverage and public health insurance programs for the poor have often ignored coverage for infertility prevention, evaluation, and treatment and may provide comprehensive healthcare insurance coverage only after a woman becomes pregnant. In addition, social programs (including family planning, contraception, sexually transmitted disease treatment, smoking cessation, and obesity prevention) that may play important roles in infertility prevention are often unavailable to poor women. This simply seems unfair.

From the perspective of the couple, infertility is often viewed as an obstacle to the fulfillment of one or both of two fundamental aspects of marriage, the creation of a family and the continuation of genetic lineage. For decades, accepting a childless family or creating a family through adoption have been seen as alternatives to the problem of infertility. But many men and women see the inability to have a child as a basic human failure, and suffer significant distress, anxiety, and depression as a result. They seek medical help in the hope that their inability to conceive can be treated with medical or surgical interventions. There are some specific medical disorders associated with infertility that can be successfully treated. In addition, medications to stimulate ovarian function and surgical interventions to correct uterine anatomic problems and fallopian tube obstruction are among the most successful treatments for women. Hormonal and antibiotic treatment and surgical interventions in men may also be curative. However, most cases of infertility are not amenable to simple treatment. In those cases, each infertile couple must acknowledge that they will not be able to overcome the problem of infertility without the use of assisted reproductive technologies. They must evaluate whether they will choose to remain childless, seek to adopt a child, or embark on a very complex and expensive odyssey that will dramatically impact their lives in order to create a child genetically linked to one or both of them.

Commentators criticize the emphasis of some individuals on the wish to have children in order to create a genetic legacy. Yet, many couples seek biologically linked children, even if only one member of the couple can successfully provide a gamete. This desire for genetic legacy seems to be a basic and powerful motivator that, since the first "test tube baby" was born in 1978, has created a large commercial industry prepared to overcome or circumvent infertility by the use of sophisticated medical technologies. Although I believe there are many problems with our present approach to regulating and paying for assisted reproductive services, I am very sympathetic to those who desire to create a genetically linked child. Creating a nurturing family in which children are loved and can grow and thrive is a laudable objective in and of itself, but the additional goal of creating a genetic legacy seems reasonable as well.

As infertility has become a more prevalent problem, creating babies with assistance of some kind results in about 6% of all births, or about 240,000 babies each year in the United States. These babies are conceived with the use of medication for ovarian stimulation or some form of assisted reproductive technology, including artificial insemination of sperm into the uterus, in vitro fertilization, and gestational surrogacy. About 50,000 babies are conceived each year in the United States with the use of in vitro fertilization (IVF): the creation of an embryo in the laboratory using one or both gametes from the infertile couple or from donors. Many commentators have been critical of assisted reproduction. Some have judged assistance with reproduction as misguided and inappropriate because it takes conception of a baby out of the personal bounds of marriage and inserts medicine and technology in areas where they do not belong. Some feminist commentators have argued that focus on infertility and its treatment degrades women and prioritizes becoming pregnant over other equally or more worthy accomplishments.

There has been much discussion about the impact of the increasing age of women at first conception on the prevalence of infertility. As women postpone marriage and creation of a family while they successfully complete educational goals and career development, they are confronted with the problem of a greater risk of infertility in their mid to late 30s when they first decide to become pregnant. There has been much debate about whether women can "have it all"—fulfillment in a career and in the creation of a family. I believe being productive in both a career and in marriage is certainly attainable, but it is difficult. It requires that young women realize that they need to plan their reproductive lives as actively as they plan their professional ones. And, it will require the society to be much more sensitive to the needs of young adults. Increasingly, we see greater flexibility in professional education, corporate and academic programs for alternative paths to success and promotion, and job-related family leave and childcare programs. These approaches can be important for many women and may help reduce infertility. Knowing that there are risk factors that increase the likelihood of infertility, young women can make thoughtful choices about prevention of sexually transmitted diseases, use of cigarettes, avoidance of environmental toxins, forestalling eating disorders and obesity, and coping with chronic stress. Young adults should have annual medical examinations to assure that their general health is good and that health problems are addressed long before they embark on creating a family.

Another approach to the problem of greater risk of infertility in women who choose to reproduce later in life is freezing eggs while young to provide a source of healthier eggs when reproduction is desired. Freezing eggs appears to be safe and effective, and young women and even children who are undergoing medical treatments that may affect egg quality and survival, such as cancer chemotherapy and gynecologic surgery, are choosing to freeze eggs or ovarian tissue for later use. Some healthy women have chosen to freeze their eggs while in their 20s and early 30s in order to ensure that they will have healthy eggs available when they decide to reproduce. Several major companies in the United States are now paying for this service for women as a benefit of employment. The companies see this as supportive of their women employees in an effort to decrease anxiety on the part of the women in their formative years with the company. The unspoken goal of this seemingly altruistic act is the inducement to decrease women employees from having earlier pregnancies that may intermittently interrupt successful careers and decrease productivity. I believe that such corporate programs are ethically justifiable, but need to be associated with a comprehensive program that supports women's health, assists with reproductive planning, and offers infertility prevention and treatment including payment for IVF as part of standard health benefits.

RELIGIOUS PERSPECTIVES ON CREATING BABIES WITH MEDICAL ASSISTANCE

Religious groups have voiced wide-ranging views on creating babies with medical assistance; within each organized religion there are disparate views on the varying approaches to overcoming infertility. There are several fundamental precepts in Catholic teaching that make almost all types of assisted reproduction unacceptable. First, since childbearing is believed to be an integral part of the marital relationship and the result of intimate sexual relations, the creation of a child in the Catholic tradition cannot include donor gametes or the creation of an embryo in a laboratory. Second, Catholic teaching strongly holds that life begins with conception.

This precept results in the conclusion that human embryos may never be destroyed as is often the case in the process of assisted reproduction. Some Catholic theologians have argued that assisted reproductive techniques utilizing gametes solely from the married couple should be permissible, since this merely extends the intimacy of the marital relationship and results in a child who is biologically related to both parents. These theologians believe it is also permissible to collect the husband's sperm from the wife's vagina after intercourse or from a condom worn during intercourse in order to insert the sperm into the wife's fallopian tube to enhance the likelihood of successfully fertilizing her egg.

Most Protestant churches approve the use of assisted reproduction but have varying views on the morality of the use of donor gametes. Many Protestant theologians believe that the introduction of a third party into the intimacy of marriage and the creation of a baby is problematic, but several Protestant groups do not unequivocally preclude the use of donor gametes. The Church of Jesus Christ of Latter Day Saints, the Mormon Church, on the other hand, generally believes that decisions concerning the use of reproductive technologies and the use of donor gametes are personal decisions to be left to the involved couple.

Islamic theologians prioritize familial lineage and the creation of children as integral parts of marriage. It is permissible, in fact encouraged, to seek medical assistance for infertile couples. If an Islamic married couple is infertile, the presumption is that the cause relates to some problem with the woman. Infertility in marriage is such a great disgrace for the man that the husband may obtain a divorce or seek a polygamous marriage in order to ensure the continuation of his genetic line. Assisted reproductive techniques with gametes from the couple are permitted. Using donor gametes is not, because Islamic law is very concerned about maintaining the purity of the familial line and the increased possibility of inadvertent consanguinity.

Orthodox Jewish tradition considers infertility a medical condition that should be aggressively evaluated and treated. Assisted reproductive technologies are permitted but destruction of embryos is more controversial. Many Jewish commentators accept the destruction of genetically abnormal embryos in the context of preimplantation genetic testing to prevent disease. Some authorities also permit the destruction of stored embryos. Clarity of genetic heritage and inadvertent consanguinity are also of great concern to Jewish theologians. Gamete donation is not precluded when it is required for the creation of a child, but Jewish law states that the resultant child should be informed about his or her true genetic heritage. Additionally, in Orthodox teaching, gamete donation should be limited to only one recipient to eliminate the potential for consanguinity.

Conservative and Reform teaching about these practices varies widely but is generally more permissive.

ETHICAL ISSUES IN IN VITRO FERTILIZATION (IVF)

IVF is the cornerstone of infertility treatment. It is the creation of embryos in a laboratory with the goal of transferring one or more embryos into a woman's uterus so that a pregnancy will occur and result in a live-born baby. Gametes for IVF are provided by one or both members of an infertile couple or by donors. Each cycle of IVF includes several steps: administering medication to artificially stimulate a woman's ovaries to develop many mature eggs in one cycle, aspiration of eggs from the ovary, obtaining fresh or frozen sperm, creating embryos in the laboratory, evaluating the quality and viability of the embryos, deciding which embryo or embryos will be transferred, inserting the embryo(s) into the uterus, monitoring the woman for pregnancy, caring for the woman and fetus throughout the pregnancy, and delivering the baby. Each of these steps is fraught with potential risks to the women and the fetus and must be successfully accomplished to result in a live-born infant.

Research in IVF

In the last 35 years, many aspects of IVF have been dramatically changed and improved through clinical innovation. Unfortunately, little, if any, research on IVF in humans has ever been funded by the National Institutes of Health (NIH) or any other United States agency. In the late 1970s around the time that Louise Brown, the first IVF baby was born in England, the United States Department of Health Education and Welfare (DHEW) [the forerunner of the present day Department of Health and Human Services (DHHS)] created an Ethics Advisory Board to review any scientifically meritorious research proposals on IVF submitted to and approved by the NIH in order to assess the moral acceptability of the proposed work. The Board approved the first such proposal and reported to the Secretary DHEW that support for IVF research was acceptable from an ethical standpoint. But the research was never funded, the Board was subsequently dissolved, and Congress explicitly precluded any research from being funded by a federal agency that involves the creation, destruction, or exposure to risk of injury or death of human embryos. Each year for the last 20 years Congress has inserted a rider to the annual budget of DHHS that explicitly states that any such activity may not be supported by federal funds under any circumstances (the Dickey-Wicker amendment, named for its congressional authors).

Since research on various aspects of IVF involves the creation and possible destruction of embryos and the exposure of embryos to various types of risk, no federally funded research studies involving human embryos have ever been performed to enhance the safety and effectiveness of IVF practice. Many questions remain about the best methods for egg retrieval; the most effective approaches to conception; the optimal media for in vitro embryo development; alternative methods for freezing, thawing, and implanting embryos; and assessment of embryo quality; to name a few. Private sources for funding this research have been inadequate because of the lack of economic benefit to the funder. Most importantly, large studies of the long-term outcomes of the babies born of IVF have never been performed. This has resulted in a field of medicine that has grown through the well intentioned work of clinical innovators without being subject to the benefits of large, well organized, federally funded clinical trials with careful institutional-review and informed-consent processes.

What is the basis of the view that federal dollars should not be used for research on IVF? At the heart of this issue is belief about the moral status of the human embryo. Without question, most embryos have the potential to develop into human beings. For some people, the potential to become a child merits conferring the same moral status to an embryo as a more developed fetus or even a child. For these individuals, even a few-day-old embryo, consisting of a small number of genetically similar but undifferentiated cells, should never be placed at risk, destroyed, or adversely affected by manipulation. They argue from a principled position that life begins at conception, when egg and sperm unite, and that all life, even potential life, is sacred and should not be destroyed. This principled view certainly deserves respect, but it seems odd to me that in a pluralistic society that a minority view should have such a great impact on others who disagree.

I have also been struck that many who hold this view of the moral status of an embryo, which precludes destruction, support allowing elderly patients who are suffering to die after withdrawal of life sustaining treatment; many also support the right of the society to invoke the death penalty for those who have committed heinous crimes. Thus, many of those who hold to the absolute prohibition of the destruction of human embryos, ostensibly based on a profound respect for all human life, are willing to permit adult members of our society to die or be killed.

Discouraging research on assisted reproduction has significant consequences. There are many unanswered questions that have serious consequences for children who will be conceived and born utilizing assisted reproduction. The prevalence of major congenital anomalies at one year of age in children born using IVF is twice that of children conceived naturally. Numerous epidemiologic studies have shown an increase in the incidence of chromosomal abnormalities and genetic imprinting errors in children conceived through IVF resulting in an increase in rare but serious genetic disorders and syndromes. Genetic imprinting is the expression of a gene contributed from one of the two parents rather than from the other. These changes in gene expression are thought to be the effect of environmental influences on genes, often referred to as an epigenetic phenomenon. Also, there are several large studies that suggest an increase in the incidence of childhood cancer in children conceived with IVF. Each of these serious problems possibly related to IVF could potentially be linked to environmental influences in the media in which the embryos are cultured; or to specific aspects of the techniques used for egg retrieval and freezing; or to embryo transfer, storage, and freezing.

Sorting out the causes of the observed increase in problems affecting children born via IVF will be difficult since the underlying causes of infertility, the age of the women receiving IVF, and the lack of a good control group for comparison studies will affect the research design and implementation. Most of the current studies on embryo development use mouse or other small animal embryos as the subjects of the research. But this animal work is insufficient to answer critical questions in humans. It remains important to perform scientifically rigorous research to understand how current laboratory methods affect human embryo development and to attempt to enhance human embryo development in vitro. When federal funding agencies provide the money, incentive, and direction for research, there is a much greater likelihood of making progress in answering such important and complex questions.

In a pluralistic society like ours, minority views, particularly those held by religious groups, should be heard and respected. But, in a nontheocratic society, should these views be determinative of what is permissible? I believe not. It seems to me that the moral status of an embryo is special because an embryo has the potential to become a person. That potentiality deserves respect and consideration in issues of clinical practice and public policy, but this does not elevate the moral status of an embryo to the status of a person bearing all those rights. For example, embryos should be respected to the extent that they should not be treated like commodities. Embryos should not be bought or sold. And they should not be part of research studies or destroyed without the permission of the gamete donors who created them. The personal values of both gamete donors should be taken into account in decisions about creation, use, storage, and destruction of embryos. Gamete donors should be permitted to decide among the various options for the disposition of an embryo: transfer to attempt the creation of a pregnancy for themselves, donation to others, immediate destruction, freezing for future decision-making about use, or donation for research. As part of the informed-consent process, a couple should understand that donation of the embryo for research will ultimately result in the destruction of the embryo. Couples should also be permitted, or even encouraged, to create embryos solely for research; this is particularly important when a couple has a known risk for producing offspring with a serious genetic disorder.

Concern for the increased prevalence of abnormalities in children conceived utilizing IVF, the unanswered scientific questions associated with techniques used in assisted reproductive techniques, and the belief that early embryos have very limited moral status, forces me to conclude that the United States should fund studies of fertility treatment and assisted reproductive techniques that might include the manipulation and possible destruction of embryos in vitro. This work and other funded clinical research studies involving IVF could have a significant impact on future children conceived through assisted reproduction.

Cost and Commercialization of IVF

Should IVF be a standard benefit in public and private health-insurance policies? The full cost of an IVF cycle in which eggs and sperm are obtained from the infertile couple and embryos created and transferred is estimated to be between $15,000 and $30,000. If donor eggs are required, the cost is significantly greater, and if previously frozen embryos are used the cost decreases by about half. This investment in the creation of a future child for an infertile couple might seem reasonable if the likelihood of success was substantial. Success rates, or so-called "take-home-baby rates," vary widely among programs and are significantly affected by the cause of the infertility, the age of the woman, and the number of cycles required to result in a live-born infant. These treatments can cost hundreds of thousands of dollars without achieving the goal of conceiving a baby who is born alive. Currently, the infertile couple pays for most of the costs.

Advertising and marketing of fertility programs is common and ubiquitous in the United States. The thoughtful consumer can review center-specific data available from the Center for Disease Control and Prevention that compares important information on techniques and outcomes among centers. However, some programs may choose to enhance outcome data by selecting healthier patients with a questionable need for IVF, or a high likelihood for success, and some centers may refuse to treat older patients or those with a low likelihood for success. These practices affect the data and make it harder for consumers to compare centers accurately when making decisions about where to seek infertility treatment. This type of gaming the system would be far less likely if IVF was covered by health insurance.

Physicians working in fertility programs, obstetrician-gynecologists with subspecialty training in reproductive endocrinology, are among the highest paid doctors in American medicine today. Their incomes are generally greater than those of their colleagues in specialties such as cardiac surgery, neurosurgery, and ophthalmology. Although the work of reproductive endocrinologists is clearly important and requires a great deal of knowledge and skill, the fees charged are completely unregulated since health insurance coverage is very limited for reproductive technologies. Thus, most couples must bear the expense of the treatments on an out-of-pocket basis. Approximately fifteen states in the United States mandate that private insurance companies include some level of health-insurance coverage for infertility treatment, but these regulations often exclude coverage for IVF. Even in states in which coverage for IVF is mandated, the total coverage may be capped at a low amount, or the number of cycles covered may be limited to one to three. Small businesses and self-insured businesses are generally exempt from such insurance mandates, and Medicaid has never covered IVF as part of family-planning services.

I believe infertility is a medical disorder that merits the provision of health insurance coverage by private and public payers. Providing health insurance for assisted reproductive techniques is not only fair, it is also likely to bring down the costs significantly and to enhance the quality of the centers. By making the centers more transparent and accountable through outside review and regulation, as has been done in many other areas in medicine, infertile patients and their future children will greatly benefit.

Since cost is such a major disincentive to infertility treatment, there are an increasing number of programs that use sliding scales for payments or even promise patients partial reimbursement if the procedures do not result in a pregnancy or a live-born baby. These programs often impose strict entrance criteria that increase the likelihood of success, and require commitments from the participants about compliance with medical recommendations about treatments and the number of embryos that will be transferred. Many commentators have criticized this practice because it may result in an increase in patients being treated with IVF who do not require such interventions, and an increase in more risky procedures including the transfer of multiple embryos to enhance the likelihood of creating a pregnancy and the delivery of a live-born baby. In addition, there has been long-standing reluctance on the part of physicians to link payment for medical treatment to guarantees of outcome. I believe that all these fee-reimbursement practices are inherently problematic, but until private and public health-insurance programs cover infertility treatments including IVF, experimenting with various payment models on a voluntary basis with clear informed-consent processes does seem acceptable.

Clinician Choice of Patients for IVF

Reproductive endocrinologists, the clinicians who evaluate and treat infertile couples and provide assisted reproductive techniques, are faced on a regular and recurring basis with deciding whether to treat a particular patient or couple. Clinicians who care for infertile couples and participate as agents in the creation of a future child must be keenly aware of the complexity of their ethical duties and obligations both to their patients and to the children who will be created. One way that clinicians discriminate against patients is through the ability to pay. Some clinicians take on a small number of no-pay patients each year, because of their concern about the unfairness of the current payment system. But should reproductive endocrinologists be allowed to discriminate in other ways, choosing which patients to treat based on age, gender orientation, marital status, medical illness, mental health, or emotional stability?

The American Medical Association (AMA) has long held that physicians, except in medical emergencies, are free to choose whom to serve. But many commentators have been concerned about the potential for physicians to discriminate against patients based on characteristics that might be unjust. Is there something special about assisted reproduction that could make some types of discrimination acceptable? Reproductive endocrinologists perform complex techniques at the request of a woman or couple that affect not only their present patient but also the children who will be born. How should reproductive endocrinologists take into account the effects of their treatment on their patients and on the children who would not have been born without their intervention?

During the early 1990s, before effective treatments were available for the prevention of human immunodeficiency virus (HIV) transmission from mother to fetus, reproductive endocrinologists routinely refused to assist women who were HIV infected to become pregnant. HIV-infected women knew that it was likely they would die, and many sought to become pregnant in order to create a legacy through the birth of a child. Since the transmission rate for HIV infection was about 25%, and since infected infants were likely to die of AIDS during infancy or carry the virus into early childhood, it was universally agreed that clinicians were justified in this discriminatory behavior. Clinicians did not argue that it was in the interests of an individual child not to be born, but rather that it was in the interests of children in general to withhold reproductive technologies that might create infants who would have a one in four chance of developing a fatal illness. At the same time, obstetricians acknowledged that the decision not to facilitate the creation of a pregnancy for women who are infertile and infected with HIV did not decrease their obligation to treat HIV-infected women who became pregnant without assistance and to support their decisions about continuing the pregnancy.

During this time, I participated in an ethics committee created by the medical school to assist the fertility program in sorting out these difficult ethical decisions. The committee discussed many cases in which clinicians were reluctant to provide assisted reproductive techniques to support the requests of patients to become pregnant. Clinicians were concerned that participation in the process of creating a pregnancy could be damaging to the woman or to the future child. We discussed cases like that of Penny Singleton and John Braithwaite (Case 1), in which an older married couple desired a child; cases of single women and lesbian couples requesting help to have a baby; cases in which a sister or a daughter volunteered to donate eggs for use by an infertile relative; and cases like Sarah Johnson (Case 3) who had serious heart or kidney disease and asked for help to have a baby. After considering the specifics of a case, a committee member would often argue that it is unethical to proceed with the treatment because it is not in the best interests of the woman or it is not in the best interests of the child because of the risks involved. We discussed each of the cases individually, trying to come up with generalizable approaches to these complex issues.

When faced with the assertion that it would be hurtful to a woman to become pregnant and carry a fetus to term because of a serious medical condition, we would first go to the literature seeking evidence about the risks of pregnancy in women with significant heart, kidney, or other diseases. We would find data about pregnancy outcomes in women with serious medical conditions who had become pregnant without medical assistance. Obstetricians reported how they, along with other medical consultants, attempted to optimize the health of the pregnant women and the outcomes of those pregnancies. Articles often concluded that outcomes of these pregnancies for the women and the fetuses varied widely.

Authors often cautioned that it would have been better for the women to forego pregnancy because of a significant incidence of maternal mortality and morbidity. But, the data also revealed excellent outcomes for some mothers and babies. Many women were willing to place themselves at considerable risk in order to become pregnant and have a baby. I was sympathetic with their desire to experience pregnancy and the possibility of giving birth to a healthy child who would live on after them. I argued that women with medical illnesses needed to be carefully evaluated to assess the individual risk of pregnancy. If the risk to the woman was reasonable and she was well informed about the possible outcomes for her and her fetus, and if she still wished to attempt to get pregnant, I counseled that it was ethically justifiable for the center to accept the patient if there was a physician willing to participate in her care. No individual physician should be coerced into participating if he or she felt that the risk to the patient was too great. As agents to the creation of a pregnancy and, therefore, as the instrument of the creation of the risky situation, reproductive endocrinologists ought to be able to refuse involvement in any case in which they believe the risk is too great even when the woman insists she wishes to take that risk for the possibility of having a baby.

When the committee discussed requests for treatment in which social concerns were evident (such as in the case of a single parent, a lesbian couple, or interfamilial egg donation), we often learned about the personal views and values of the clinicians and we considered whether refusal to participate in the care was idiosyncratic or should be generalized to the level of a policy of the center. When reproductive endocrinologists consider which patients they wish to accept, the interests of the child who will be born are relevant; but the race, sexual orientation, or age of the couple seeking help are rarely, if ever, appropriate criteria to justify refusal of care.

We made distinctions between those patient requests that were reasonable and should be accepted by the center, if an individual physician agreed, and those that were ethically troubling and should not be accepted. The committee focused on known risks of harm to the woman or child as the major criteria for rejecting patients, not social circumstances. I believe physicians are moral agents and must be responsible for their personal actions in caring for patients; and I agree with the AMA assertion that physicians in nonemergent situations are free to choose whom to serve. But I am appalled when physicians use patient social or behavioral characteristics to justify refusing to treat a patient rather than medically relevant issues. Early in its existence, our program accepted single women, gay and lesbian couples, and many other individuals and couples who were rejected by other programs. We justified our decisions by using the literature that revealed that children in loving families did well regardless of the age or sexual orietnation of their parents, or even if there was only one parent.

I believe it makes sense to create policies based on objective medical criteria about which groups of patients will or will not be accepted for treatment. The center may wish to reserve the option to accept or reject an individual patient under extraordinary circumstances, but clear policies can be very helpful in preventing blatant discrimination. Because psychological factors are relevant in decision-making about whether to accept an individual patient or couple for treatment, programs should use psychological evaluations to help assess the motivation and stability of a patient or couple and their ability to cope with the stresses of assisted reproduction and the responsibilities of parenting. This practice has become universally accepted and can be helpful to both the patients and the clinicians.

Gamete Donation

Gamete donation is a critical and important part of infertility treatment. Although some IVF cycles can utilize gametes obtained from the infertile couple, many infertile couples require gamete donation to overcome infertility. Some religious groups discourage gamete donation, whereas other groups tolerate or even encourage it. Reproductive endocrinologists must be aware of the ethical and legal problems inherent in gamete donation. Some states have specific laws about the screening of potential donors but most reproductive technology programs must create their own standards. These standards include concern about the health of the donor, the quality of the gametes, reproductive and fertility history, genetic history, and age. Donors are required to be of legal age to consent to the donation and are often screened for sexually transmitted diseases with questionnaires about sexual history and symptoms, as well as blood tests for syphilis, hepatitis B, and HIV. Since there is a significant incubation period for HIV antibodies to become positive after exposure, donated sperm is generally frozen for six months and donors retested for HIV antibodies. Although eggs can be frozen, fresh egg donation is more commonly used in IVF. Therefore, infectious disease testing and screening must be accomplished before donation and increases the risk (although small) that the egg will carry HIV.

Genetic screening of donors generally includes a thorough family history, as well as carrier screening for those recessive genetic disorders that might be prevalent in the donor's ethnic background. Donors are often rejected due to family histories that include alcoholism or other substance abuse, autism, severe mental illness, and homosexuality. Questionnaires and interviews are the methods used to determine family and personal history and are, of course, subject to the honesty and knowledge of the potential donor, placing the infertile couple at significant risk that donated gametes could contain genetic abnormalities that might affect the future child.

Should gamete donors be compensated or should this be an altruistic act like organ donation? Sperm donation is not a risky procedure and is compensated modestly. Egg donation is a far more complex and risky procedure. Eggs are sometimes donated by women undergoing egg retrieval for their own infertility treatment who produce "extra" eggs, or from relatives or friends of the infertile couple, or from healthy women recruited by the fertility program. Many view the recruitment of and substantial payment to healthy young women, often college students who have never been pregnant, to be ethically problematic. Donation is inherently risky even in healthy women, and the levels of compensation are considered by many to be an undue inducement. Women require medication to stimulate ovulation and anesthesia for egg retrieval. Each of these steps has significant risks and the potential for long-term health consequences to the donor. Advertising for donors often takes place in college and local newspapers and via the Internet and social media sites. Compensation of many thousands of dollars is not unusual. The sheer amount of money offered for donation and the risks of the medications and procedures make this practice ethically troubling. Yet, without donor eggs many couples will be unable to overcome infertility.

The use of friends and family members as egg donors can overcome some of these ethical concerns, but may create others. Donation by those close to the infertile couple rarely is compensated except for the medical costs of the actual donation. However, gamete donation may create the potential for conflict after the birth of the child. Despite the best of intentions, as the child grows up, tensions may develop about parenting issues, and confusion may develop about maternal rights and responsibilities between the biologic and gestational mothers. Merely informing the child about the existence of the relative who is his biologic mother does not resolve this problem. The child may experience significant harm from parenting conflicts and become confused and upset by the feuding adults.

As the practice of IVF and egg donation has become commonplace in the Untied States, a few commentators have sought to preclude all donation based on ethical grounds. More commonly, the current approach to anonymous compensated donation is justified by ensuring that donors are given sufficient information and time to make a truly informed choice. There has been great concern about the amount of compensation and the potential for that incentive to result in women placing themselves at repeated risk through multiple donations. Although programs can limit the number of times an individual may donate and can ask potential donors whether they have donated before to other programs, there are no real safeguards against a woman donating multiple times in various programs and placing herself at increasing risk with each donation.

I believe that women can and should be permitted to make the decision about whether and how often they will donate eggs to infertility programs even though there is substantial risk inherent in this procedure. I would limit the level of payment to make it reasonable compensation for the time and risk, and would cap compensation to reduce the incentive for multiple repeat donations. In the case of anonymous donation, informed consent should also include a reminder that egg donation will likely result in the donor having genetically linked children with whom there will be no relationship, and that any of her own future children will likely have half siblings who they will not know.

Should infertile couples be concerned about consanguinity in their future grandchildren? Consanguinity in the future is an inadvertent risk of IVF with donated gametes. Children who have been conceived from gametes from the same donor may develop a relationship and ultimately reproduce resulting in a consanguineous child subject to a substantial genetic risk of recessive disorders. Although the risks of two children conceived from the same donor meeting and developing a relationship are small, it warrants some concern. An effort to limit the number of babies created from one donor seems reasonable and appropriate. Sperm or egg donation from an individual donor should be limited to a small number, perhaps ten, in order to make consanguinity extremely unlikely. Unfortunately, there are few laws in the United States that regulate this practice. Clinicians are obligated to ensure that their patients are protected by monitoring the practices of sperm banks with which they are associated and by limiting the number of egg donations from any individual woman.

Should gamete donation be anonymous? Another way to deal with the problem of consanguinity is to eliminate anonymity in gamete donation. There is increasing advocacy by donor-conceived individuals to make gamete donation "open," similar to the open-adoption movement. Donors would no longer be anonymous and children conceived with a donor gamete would be informed of their status and encouraged to communicate with and meet their genetic parent. At the current time, gamete donation is generally anonymous and many children are unaware that they were conceived with donor gametes. Some children who have been informed about their status seek additional information about their genetic parent and with the help of rudimentary data from sperm banks or donor egg programs can sometimes utilize the Internet and social media sites to find their genetic parent. The identification of a genetic parent can be very important to a child's identity and provide insight into the background of their physical appearance, personality, and interests. Additionally, there is a great deal of medical and genetic information that is unavailable if the donor is anonymous. As knowledge of familial history of illness becomes increasingly important in medical practice, there will be more pressure to make donors known or to at least provide substantial medical and genetic information in an anonymous manner to children born from donor gametes.

Children conceived with donor gametes may also benefit from knowing about diseases and conditions that other children conceived with gametes from that same donor may have acquired over time. There are several proposed ways to assure that such information is made available. Some of these models maintain donor anonymity, whereas others preclude it. Web-based information systems with continual update of medical information from donors and recipients can increase the level of information available to recipients. These programs can work regardless of whether or not the donor remains anonymous.

Open adoption has become increasingly common in the United States and most experts in child development recommend informing adopted children of their status. Adopted children who have not been told frequently learn inadvertently of their status during childhood from a parent, relative, or family friend. Adoption is often difficult to keep secret because of the lack of a pregnancy associated with the appearance of a new baby in the family. Pediatricians and child psychologists believe that keeping adoption a secret can be very harmful to the development of attachment and trust if a child learns inadvertently that he is not genetically related to his parents. In contrast, the use of a donor gamete to create a pregnancy can easily be kept secret from the future child and from virtually everyone else if the couple wishes to maintain the secret.

I am sympathetic to those children who wish to know more about their genetic parents but I am not convinced that at the present time recommending open donation in all cases of gamete donation is in the best interest of the children. Some families may wish to keep this secret and may feel strongly that it is not in the best interest of their child to know. I think we need to experiment with several Web-based models that permit anonymous donation of gametes but require continual update of medical and genetic information from the donor that can be made available to the child and the family. We should also be experimenting with open and transparent donation, with the expectation that the infertile couple will inform their child of his or her status and encourage the development of a relationship between the donor and the child. Research studies that collect data on the impact of these models on all stakeholders are crucial to determine public policy in the future. In all cases of gamete donation, there is a need for clarity about the legal responsibilities of the gamete donor vis-à-vis future support of the child. Gamete donation programs will not be possible if donors are at risk for financial support of the future child. State laws and all parties must be clear about what, if any, responsibilities are attached to the altruistic act of gamete donation.

Gamete Storage and Disposition

For decades, sperm have been successfully frozen, stored, and thawed for use in reproduction. Recently, freezing and storage of eggs and ovarian tissue have become standard practice in assisted reproduction. Gametes can be frozen and stored for future use by an individual or donated for use by others. Gametes should be considered the "property" of the donor until such time as the donor voluntarily gives them to a program for others to use for procreation or for research purposes.

For young girls who are facing chemotherapy and radiation for the treatment of cancer or other diseases, pediatric oncologists have recommended freezing and storing gametes for future use. At birth, a woman's ovaries contain all the eggs she will ever produce. Chemotherapy, even if successful in curing a disease, often results in significant ovarian failure and infertility. Ovarian tissue can be obtained by minimally invasive laparoscopic surgery from the child before cancer treatment commences, frozen for storage, and reimplanted into the girl after she is cancer free and desires to consider reproduction. Similarly, sperm or testicular tissue from boys facing cancer treatment or testicular removal may be frozen and stored for future use. Sperm are replaceable if testicular function is normal but many diseases and their treatments make the creation of new sperm impossible.

Many commentators have questioned whether children should be subjected to a surgical procedure that requires anesthesia in order to preserve gametes for possible use in reproduction many years later. Infertility is often very upsetting to many couples, and maintaining genetic lineage is felt to be important. Enabling a young cancer patient the option of creating a genetically linked offspring justifies the minimally invasive procedure that is required to preserve the tissue. However, there is a need to gather additional data on the outcomes of the children produced using these techniques. Since many cancers are genetically determined, will future offspring be more likely to develop cancer? Will freezing of tissues result in a greater incidence of birth defects, prematurity, or growth restriction in future children? To answer these questions, longitudinal studies will be required and there will be a need to examine the best ways to approach the child and family about participation in such research.

I believe these practices should be encouraged and that research should be funded to ensure the safety and efficacy of the procedures. All such research is voluntary and should require the consent of the parents and the assent of the child if developmentally appropriate. Although we are learning more about these practices through research, there is also a need to deal with the issue of the disposition of the gametes. Sadly, the children who donate the tissues may die from the cancer. The consent of the tissue or gamete donor should be required for any decision that results in a reproductive use of the tissue. Even though the consent of the parents was required for storage of the tissue, the fact that these gametes are uniquely related to the child should preclude the parents from permitting the use of the gametes for procreation. Gametes should not be treated as commodities that can be bought or sold and only the person who created the gametes should be permitted to decide if another human being would be created with these tissues. If the child dies before becoming capable of independent decision-making, the gametes should never be used for reproduction. Without specific permission, the grieving parents or the loving fiancé of the deceased donor should not be permitted to utilize the gametes for reproduction, even if justified as an attempt to create a meaningful legacy for their lost loved one.

This conclusion is based primarily on a profound respect for the gamete donor as responsible for all reproductive choices concerning his or her own gametes. Concern for the interests of the children who might be born from reproductive use of the gametes is less critical in my analysis, but also relevant. During the grieving process, many families are overwhelmed by the acute loss and might wish to bring some aspect of that loved person back into the family. Having stored gametes from the lost loved one might be seen as a way to make this wish a reality. But the complex and conflicted nature of the family's motivation and the potential for serious psychological problems for the future child who results from the stored gametes make this an unwise decision that should not be permitted. Parents should be empowered to consent to research with the stored gametes of their deceased child, as long as there will be no attempt at the creation of a child. All gametes and tissues from a deceased child should be destroyed if the family has declined to donate the gametes for research.

Embryos

There are hundreds of thousands of frozen embryos stored in fertility clinics around the country. The stewardship of these embryos is a great responsibility. Each embryo should be afforded the respect of being uniquely identified as related to those persons who created it. There have been errors in identification of stored embryos and subsequent transfer of those embryos into the wrong women, resulting in the births of children not intended by those who stored the embryos and not related to those who become their parents. It is important that information on the identity of each embryo be conscientiously maintained so that the person or couple who have consented to the storage of the embryo can be confident in their disposition. We have discussed the ethical justification for the storage and disposition of embryos including the potential for research and destruction of embryos. Importantly, those who have created and stored the embryo should each be involved in its disposition.

Anonymous gamete donors cede responsibility for the future fate of their gametes when an embryo is created. Before donation, anonymous gamete donors should be informed that embryos created from their gametes may immediately be transferred into a uterus in an attempt to create a pregnancy or, alternatively, may be frozen for future use. The donors should also be aware that future uses for frozen embryos include donation to other couples for procreation, or to institutions for research, and the possibility of destruction. Donors should be fully informed and should consent to all of these possible uses or they should consent only to certain specific uses of their gametes. Each fertility program needs to assure respect for these choices or only accept donations that allow for all potential uses of the gametes.

When couples choose to store excess embryos, the informed-consent process should clearly explain the responsibility of the couple to maintain current contact information with the clinic and to accept that, if the embryos are abandoned, after a certain period of time they will be destroyed. The fertility program has some level of responsibility to try to locate couples who have not maintained contact, but after due diligence, the clinic has the right to destroy excess embryos.

There have been many cases in which one of the members of a couple who has stored embryos seeks to utilize an embryo without the informed consent of the other member of the couple. This situation often transpires after the death of one spouse or the divorce of the couple. Respect for the reproductive potential of the embryo and the right of each person to determine their future reproductive choices mandates that an embryo not be utilized by one member of the couple who created it without the consent of the other. Many legal cases have affirmed this general principle. And, analogous to the discussion on the posthumous use of stored gametes, embryos should not be used for procreation without the explicit permission of each of the members of the couple under whose stewardship the embryos were created. This is a bit more complicated ethically and legally if the embryo has a donated gamete and is only linked genetically to the living member of the couple. Nonetheless, the process by which the embryo was created and stored was a shared decision by the couple who became the stewards for the embryo and should require the consent of each member of the couple to determine disposition.

Preimplantation Genetic Diagnosis

Over the last 25 years, IVF programs have developed the capacity to provide genetic testing of a single cell from an early embryo in order to determine if the embryo is affected with a chromosomal abnormality or single gene mutation. This technique is called preimplantation genetic diagnosis (PGD). The extraction of a single cell from an embryo in the early stage of development without negative consequence is possible because each of the cells is undifferentiated and has the full potential to develop into the future child. PGD has also been used for the determination of cancer susceptibility, risk of adult-onset diseases such as Alzheimer's Disease, and sex selection to avoid X-linked disorders, as well as identification of an appropriate hematopoietic stem cell donor for an affected sibling. Resultant pregnancy rates and the outcome of the children after PGD seem comparable to IVF without embryo biopsy. PGD has been very controversial because it often results in the destruction of unwanted normal or affected embryos, and permits the selection of embryos to be implanted based on the presence or absence of specific genetic traits.

Those who oppose IVF because of the potential to manipulate, adversely affect, or destroy embryos are certainly opposed to PGD. Those who accept the new reproductive technologies as innovative approaches that expand options for infertile couples generally accept PGD, but some may have concerns about the justification of specific uses of PGD or intentional selection of specific embryos for implantation.

Should PGD be used for sex selection? When PGD is used for gender selection not related to X-linked disease, it is very controversial. Many commentators oppose the use of PGD for sex selection if it is unrelated to disease prevention. Some feminists argue that any use of PGD for sex selection unrelated to disease prevention should be prohibited because the practice has the potential to demean women in a culture that is likely to prioritize male children. It is also feared that familial and cultural preference for male offspring and limits on total numbers of children permitted in certain cultures will result in a significant disparity in sex ratio that will result in many negative consequences. Some, however, accept sex selection through PGD for family "balancing," the practice of determining the gender of subsequent children after having one or more children of the same sex. They justify their belief by reference to the suggested benefits of being exposed during development to siblings of the other sex, and sympathy for couples who have always wished to parent a child of that particular sex.

I believe that use of PGD is a reasonable option for prevention of a known genetic disease, embryo screening in the face of a strong family history of a genetic disorder, and gender balancing in families who have two or three children of the same sex. This last use is quite controversial but, in recent years, is being requested more frequently. Any clinician who does not wish to use his or her knowledge and skills for gender selection, preferring to use PGD only for disease prevention, should not be criticized.

The use of PGD to ensure the birth of a sibling to provide a stem cell transplant for a child with a serious hematological disorder remains controversial. Betty and Jesus Morales in Case 2 seek IVF and PGD to create a matched sibling to help their son Pablo who is suffering from Hodgkin's lymphoma. Stem cell transplantation utilizing umbilical cord blood or bone marrow has become the standard approach to treatment of many hematologic disorders. For some of these disorders, the best results are found when stem cells are very closely matched between donor and recipient. Unaffected siblings or other close relatives are generally the best choice for stem cell donation. In the United States today, there are public banks of umbilical cord blood and bone marrow that can be used for stem cell transplantation. Unfortunately, affected children who are minorities, like Pablo Morales often do not find close enough matches in public banks or among their relatives. In this situation, families have no options to help their seriously ill child other than to create a sibling who might be able to donate stem cells for transplantation. The chance of an unselected sibling being both unaffected by the genetic disorder and matched for critical markers of compatibility required for transplant success is about 1 in 5. The use of PGD dramatically increases the chance for success since the selected embryo will be both unaffected and closely matched.

Commentators have argued that the new child, so conceived, has been created as a means to assist the affected child, and not out of a genuine desire for another child as an end in itself. Betty and Jesus Morales were not planning to have another child since they were somewhat overwhelmed by Pablo's illness and his constant need for doctor visits and hospitalizations. But they decided to try to help their son through IVF and PGD.

Should they be criticized for their motivation for creating a new child? Pablo's doctors also explained to the Moraleses that there is a considerable risk that the stem cell transplant obtained from the umbilical cord blood from the new baby will not be successful in curing Pablo's lymphoma. Thus they run the risk, if the transplant is unsuccessful, that Pablo will die and they may be left with ambivalent feelings about the child they created to rescue him.

The Moraleses fully understood the risks, were sure they would love their new baby regardless of the outcome for Pablo, and went forward with egg retrieval and IVF with the creation of ten embryos. PGD found only one embryo that was both unaffected and a close match for Pablo. The embryo was transferred to Betty's uterus and resulted in a successful pregnancy. Umbilical cord blood was obtained at birth and hematologic stem cells were harvested and stored for transplant to Pablo. After preparing Pablo with aggressive chemotherapy, the stem cell transplant was performed and resulted in successful remission of the tumor. At age 6, Pablo is a healthy boy and loves to play with his one year old brother, Angel.

It seems reasonable to me that a loving family would take the risks that Betty and Jesus undertook. They would hope to have the best of all possible outcomes, while being prepared to accept the destinies of each child and embrace them in their loving family regardless of what happened. An argument could be made that Betty and Jesus had an ethical obligation to their affected son, Pablo, to do all they reasonably could to help him, including creating Angel, with the hope that the stem cell transplant would be successful. I share this view and would encourage any couple in similar circumstances to consider all their options including IVF and PGD, but I would not unduly coerce any couple to make such a choice. I believe that any couple who is so considerate of the needs of their existing child that they would go through the entire process of IVF and PGD is likely to display that same love and caring for their new child and to cherish that child independent of its utility as a donor.

GESTATIONAL SURROGACY

In Case 3, Sarah and Fred Johnson seek the help of a gestational surrogate in order to accomplish their goal of having a baby. Surrogate parenting is a social arrangement in which a woman provides the service of becoming pregnant and delivering a baby for a couple she is not related to. This arrangement generally separates genetic and gestational aspects of childbearing and includes an agreement by the surrogate to relinquish all maternal rights shortly after birth. Gestational surrogacy is generally used when a woman who wishes to have a family is unable to become pregnant for various reasons related to her health. Should our society permit this practice? Should we encourage it?

Physicians treating Sarah determined that it was very dangerous for her to be pregnant since the physiologic changes that occur during pregnancy would place her at considerable personal risk, and might result in a baby born preterm or small for gestational age due to intrauterine growth restriction. Sarah and Fred chose to use a donor egg and created an embryo utilizing Fred's sperm. The embryo was then transferred into the surrogate for gestation.

Gestational surrogacy involves an agreement between the surrogate and the intended parents. Surrogates are generally women of low socioeconomic status who have been pregnant previously. Intended parents are generally sufficiently affluent to be able to afford IVF, and can provide the funds to pay for the surrogate's services. Agreements between the parties spell out the surrogate's obligations to attend all prenatal health care visits, to accept any needed tests or medications during pregnancy, to eat well, to not take drugs or drink alcohol, and perhaps, most importantly, to relinquish maternal rights to the child shortly after birth. The intended parents compensate the surrogate for her efforts and pay all expenses of the health care. There generally is a written contract that is signed between the parties. Many contracts include paragraphs about unexpected events like the promise to abort the fetus if medical testing determines that the child will have a serious genetic or anatomic abnormality, and the obligation of the intended patents to take responsibility for the child after birth regardless of the child's condition.

Fred and Sarah Johnson encountered such an unexpected event when at the time of delivery, the surrogate refused to relinquish maternal rights to the child. Even though she was genetically unrelated to the child, after the birth she was overwhelmed with grief at the thought of giving away the baby she had carried for nine months.

The legal status of gestational surrogates and the ability to enforce contracts between surrogates and intended parents varies widely among states in the United States and throughout the world. Enforcing agreements or even contracts that obligate individuals in the areas of pregnancy and adoption are very controversial because of the rights and interests of the child who is involved. Should the person who gestates and delivers the child be considered the "mother" with all legal rights and responsibilities? Should the genetic make up of the child play any role in determining parenthood? What rights does the genetic father have in such a case?

There are many issues that need resolution when parental status and child custody questions arise after gestational surrogacy. Each case is different and state laws vary widely, so it is uncertain how a court would view the issues raised in a specific gestational surrogacy case. The interests of the child, and the fundamental constitutional right to procreative liberty of the intended parents makes some commentators believe that surrogacy contracts are protected and should be enforced. Others see surrogacy contracts in the realm of commercial transactions that are illegal, like baby selling. As courts have reviewed these cases, the woman who carries and delivers the baby is generally considered the mother of the child and granted all maternal rights. The genetic father can claim his rights and may seek custody of the child. The intended mother who is neither the genetic mother nor the birth mother would have very little standing in the custody dispute.

From the perspective of the interests of the child who is born after gestational surrogacy, there is a need to promptly establish parental status and custody in order to provide a stable, secure, and nurturing environment for the child. If surrogacy is to be permitted, it is vitally important to create laws and social structures that protect the interests of the children who will be born. Some commentators believe that the interests of children are best served by laws that strictly regulate the practice of surrogacy and enforce the contracts. They suggest that the surrogate is being paid for her gestational services, not for the child she delivers, and she should be obligated to relinquish her rights to the child at birth.

Some critics of surrogacy maintain that separating genetic and gestational components of birth is immoral because it separates conception and gestation of a child from the sanctity of marriage. Others argue that surrogacy amounts to baby selling and that, if surrogacy is permitted, the interests of the children cannot be protected. Some feminists argue that surrogacy degrades women by defining them as vessels that can be purchased or rented for the creation of children. Commentators also voice concerns about children who are born preterm or with disabling conditions might be abandoned by both the gestational mother and the intended parents.

I am very sympathetic to the desire of an infertile couple to have a genetically related child to at least one member of the pair, when the woman is unable for health reasons to become pregnant or carry a fetus. Surrogacy is that couple's only hope for a genetically related child. Although I believe that surrogacy should be permitted, I do not believe contracts should be enforceable. I do not believe women should be forced to have an abortion under any circumstances, nor should they be coerced to accept unwanted tests or treatments that place them at significant risk. I would hope that all surrogates are willing to relinquish their maternal rights shortly after birth, but I believe that carrying a baby through a pregnancy is such a profoundly important experience that it merits the legal designation of mother of that newborn. This would require that the law support the surrogate if she does not wish to relinquish the child for adoption by the intended couple.

If contracts are unenforceable, everyone involved is at risk. This may drive some infertile couples to reassess the importance of genetic linkage to their child, and to seek adoption as an alternative to surrogacy. Gestational surrogacy has worked well in most cases and has resulted in children who are loved and nurtured by their intended parents. Nonetheless, from the child's perspective, there are great risks if the surrogate decides that she wishes to keep her baby or if the intended parents reject the child because of a serious medical problem at birth. I believe courts should support the gestational mother's right to not relinquish custody of the child, and the genetic father's right to seek custody. This would reflect the type of process that goes on in a divorce proceeding. When there is conflict, the court should make "best interest" assessments about the future of the child as soon after birth as possible. For those children with serious disorders, the intended parents should not be allowed to disregard their responsibilities to the child after birth and should be held accountable similar to other parents of disabled newborns.

FINAL THOUGHTS

Infertility is a serious and growing problem in the United States. We have learned a great deal in the past 35 years about how assisted reproductive technologies can be used to help infertile couples fulfill their desire to have children. There remain many scientific, clinical, legal, ethical, and policy issues that require our attention and deliberation. From my perspective, the key ethical question that needs to be addressed when we analyze any of the issues associated with these approaches to creating babies is what do we owe the future children who will be created utilizing assisted reproductive technologies?

We owe the future children federal research funding to ensure that the techniques and procedures used in assisted reproduction are as safe and effective as possible. There is a need for additional research on optimizing embryo development in vitro and identifying embryos that are most likely to result in a healthy fetus and a successful pregnancy. More comprehensive epidemiologic data are needed to determine which processes are associated with healthy or abnormal short- and long-term outcomes for the women and the children.

Clinical practices should be modified to eliminate the increasing number of twin pregnancies that are associated with assisted reproduction. Assisted reproductive technologies account for about 1.2% of all live births in the United States but 16% of the twins. Over the past decade, through voluntary compliance with generally accepted standards in the field, the number of triplet and higher-order multiple pregnancies has decreased dramatically in the United States but the number of twin pregnancies has risen. This is due to the common practice of the transfer of two embryos at the time of an IVF procedure.

Although many infertile couples consider the birth of twins to be a highly desirable outcome, over 60% of twins are born preterm, at less than 37 weeks of gestation. Prematurity has serious short- and long-term consequences for the child, and even babies born "late preterm," at 34–37 weeks gestation, have increased mortality and morbidity as compared to full-term infants. Couples may wish to have twins because this allows them to have two children and "complete" their desired family with only one pregnancy. This is sometimes due to the desire to avoid the risks to the woman of a second pregnancy especially if she is in her mid- or late-30s. But choosing to have twins is more likely due to the way we pay for assisted reproductive treatments. The cost is high and there is limited insurance coverage for these procedures, leading many couples to choose multiple embryo transfers. Current programs in the United States, and elsewhere that include only single-embryo transfer are reported to result in excellent pregnancy and "take home baby" rates, without the increased incidence of twins. Recognition of the interests of the children who will be conceived requires that society require payment for reproductive technologies through public- and private-health-insurance coverage for infertility treatments, and that it develop regulations to encourage single-embryo transfers.

Helping infertile couples create babies is a laudable use of medical expertise. But children who will be conceived with the help of assisted reproductive technologies deserve more careful and thoughtful attention to their interests as the field grows and develops.

ADDITIONAL READINGS

Johnston J, Gusmano MK. Why we should all pay for fertility treatment. *Hastings Center Report*, 2013; 43:18–21.

Robertson JA, Kahn JP, Wagner JE, Conception to obtain hematopoietic stem cells. *Hastings Center Report*, 2002; 32:34–40.

Patrizio P, Caplan AL. Ethical issues surrounding fertility preservation in cancer patients. *Clin Obstet Gynecol*, 2010; 53:717–726.

The New York State Task Force on Life and the Law. Assisted Reproductive Technologies. New York, NY:1998.

The New York State Task Force on Life and the Law. Surrogate Parenting. New York, NY:1988.

Baruch S, Kaufman D, Hudson KL. Genetic testing of embryos: Practices and perspectives of US in vitro fertilization clinics. *Fertil Steril*, 2008; 89:1053–1058.

Schieve LA, Meikle SF, Ferre C, et al. Low and very low birth weight in infants conceived with use of assisted reproductive technology. *N Engl J Med*, 2002; 346:731–737.

Hansen M, Kurinczuk JJ, Bower C, Webb S. The risk of major birth defects after intracytoplasmic sperm injection and in vitro fertilization. *N Engl J Med*, 2002; 346:725–730.

McLernon DJ, Harrild K, Bergh C, et al. Clinical effectiveness of single versus double embryo transfer: meta-analysis of individual patient data from randomized trials. *BMJ*, 2010; 341:1–13, online first *BMJ*.

Institute of Medicine. Behrman RE, Butler AS (eds), *Preterm Birth: Causes, Consequences, and Prevention*. Washington DC: National Academies Press: 2006.

CHAPTER 3
Ethical Issues in Giving Birth to a Baby

Case 1

Mary Brightman is a 37-year-old attorney who is 36 weeks into her first pregnancy. She has been very healthy throughout the pregnancy and has been able to work diligently as a fourth-year associate focusing on corporate law in a major New York City firm. Mary read all the books that explain how to have a healthy pregnancy and a good birth. She prepared a birth plan that she hoped to share with her obstetrician at her next prenatal visit; it describes how she would like her labor and delivery to unfold. The plan includes specific instructions to assure that the birth is as natural as possible: a quiet labor-delivery room with dim lighting and a closed door, no visitors other than Mary's husband Tom and the doula that Mary hired for support, no doctors-in-training or medical students, no fetal monitor, no intravenous, no epidural or drugs for pain management, and immediate access to the baby after delivery for skin to skin contact and initiation of breast feeding. But Mary has just learned that her primary client, a very large multinational corporation, is going to acquire their largest competitor in a hostile takeover that will occur in four weeks. She is terribly distressed because she knows that successfully assisting her client with this acquisition will almost certainly assure her future as a partner in her law firm and that missing this opportunity is likely to result in her not making partner for the foreseeable future or possibly being let go from the firm. Mary explores her options and a few days later, at the 37-week prenatal visit informs her obstetrician that because she is now at term, she would like to have a scheduled cesarean delivery as soon as possible so that she can return to work in a few weeks.

Tanya Chambers is a 25-year-old woman in her first pregnancy. At 40-weeks gestation her membranes ruptured and she presented to the hospital in early labor. Tanya received antibiotics and labor progressed slowly. After 18 hours of ruptured membranes Tanya was noted to have a fever of 39°C (102.2° F) and the fetal heart was beating very rapidly with significant decelerations not associated with contractions. The nurses and doctors were concerned for both Tanya and her baby and began to prepare for an emergency cesarean delivery. After the obstetrician explained the seriousness of the problem to Tanya and explained the need for a cesarean delivery, Tanya admitted that she was frightened by the prospect of surgery and refused to consent. She said that her mother had five babies with no cesarean deliveries and that she was certain she would be able to delivery this baby if given a bit more time. The doctors explained that the baby might die from an overwhelming infection, and that Tanya might be very sick or die as well, if they did not perform the cesarean delivery as soon as possible. Tanya continued to refuse to consent to the surgery.

Throughout history, women, their partners, and their health professionals have realized that there are serious medical and ethical issues involved in being pregnant and giving birth to a child. Most pregnant women envision going into labor and having a vaginal birth as the natural and best culmination of being pregnant. Pregnancy, labor, and delivery are natural events, but they are also potentially fraught with risk to both the woman and fetus, and sometimes require important choices on the part of the woman and her healthcare professionals. Every pregnant woman wants a good birth, but a good birth is not only a birth in which both the mother and baby turn out healthy. Women anticipate the birth process with high expectations not just for a good outcome, but also for a joyous experience that sets the tone for a loving relationship with the baby. A good birth, then, is one that is consistent with the views and values of the woman and her partner, and fulfills all their hopes and wishes.

In America today, many physicians and other healthcare professionals participate in the care of a pregnant woman and her fetus, assisting in planning for labor and delivery, and possibly intervening in the birth process. What are the ethical obligations of healthcare providers to a pregnant woman and to her fetus who will be born? What are the ethical obligations of a pregnant woman to her fetus who will be born as a viable child?

Healthcare professionals clearly have beneficence based obligations to pregnant women to protect and promote their medical and health-related interests. They also have autonomy-based obligations to respect the decisions of the pregnant woman as an adult with the capacity to make health-care choices for themselves. These ethical obligations are similar to those encountered in any clinical transaction with a capacitated adult. However, because pregnancy is such a unique experience, many obstetric ethicists argue that health professionals have a second set of ethical obligations to their pregnant patients that includes promoting a woman's values and preferences as she defines them relating to the pregnancy. These obligations require that health professionals elicit the patient's values and preferences regarding the circumstances of how she will be treated in labor and delivery and, unless there are compelling reasons to the contrary, implement her wishes. These various ethical obligations rarely come in conflict, but when they do, it is generally because the health professional views the woman's preferences about labor and delivery will impact negatively on the health and well-being of her developing fetus and the child it will become.

Virtually any physician who cares for a fetus who will become a child feels beneficence-based moral obligations to protect and promote the health-related interests of that fetus. Some professionals feel that these obligations are less important than their ethical obligations to the pregnant woman, but nonetheless, all professionals feel conflicted when they perceive that their actions or a decision by a pregnant woman may result in harm to a fetus who is destined to become a child.

Some commentators argue that these ethical conflicts can be resolved by clarifying the moral status of the fetus. I disagree. Whether one believes that a fetus has independent moral status equivalent to an already born child, or that a fetus has evolving moral status with increasing gestational age, or that a fetus has no independent moral status, if the decision has been made to bring the fetus to viability with the goal of delivering a baby, the fetus merits our concern. In situations in which the health-related interests of the woman and the fetus are not identical, the professional faces a serious conflict that needs to be resolved. Such conflicts are not common in obstetrics but they do exist and require careful consideration. Uniquely in obstetrics, when a fetus becomes viable, a single clinician is treating two patients with independent and potentially conflicting interests. Whatever the belief about the moral status of the developing fetus, when a fetus is viable and can survive outside the uterus, it clearly becomes a patient, and generates ethical obligations on the part of the clinician to act to enhance its health-related interests. These obligations are not unlimited and must be balanced against the clinician's ethical obligations to respect the autonomy of the woman and to promote her health-related interests as well.

Pregnant women also have beneficence-based ethical obligations to their fetuses who will become children. We expect that a pregnant woman will behave in a manner that promotes her own interests and the interests of her fetus by not drinking alcohol, not smoking, and not taking illicit drugs. We expect that a pregnant woman will consider not only her own interests, but also those of her fetus when making health-related decisions concerning her pregnancy and delivery. A woman's beneficence-based obligations to her fetus are not unlimited. We should not ask women to ignore their own interests when making decisions that affect their fetuses, but we do ask them to take fetal interests into consideration.

Pediatricians and neonatologists, newborn specialists, are frequently consulted in the latter part of pregnancy when obstetric professionals and pregnant women need to make hard choices about treatment for health-related problems that affect the pregnancy and could result in early delivery of the fetus. Neonatologists come to these discussions with perspectives that may differ significantly from those of obstetricians. Neonatologists see their patient as the newborn. Virtually all commentators believe that a newborn has independent moral status worthy of respect. Thus, birth, with the transition from intrauterine to extrauterine existence, brings with it a clear set of beneficence-based obligations to the newborn. Both the clinicians and the new mother have a duty to promote the interests of the vulnerable infant. Although parents and clinicians may have differing views of what constitutes the best interest of a newborn, resolving these value conflicts is quite different from the weighing of choices for a fetus. Although all decisions for an infant clearly affect the parents, and although pediatricians respect parents as integral to decision-making for children, in considering physician obligations to a newborn, there are no autonomy-based obligations to the parents. This is because the parents are not patients of the neonatologist and the decision for the newborn does not directly affect the health-related interests of the parents. Parents are surrogate decision-makers for their children who cannot make autonomous decisions for themselves.

Our society gives great deference to parents in making choices in a wide range of decisions concerning the health and well-being of their children. This deference is consistent with our belief that parents are almost always the best arbiters of the interests of their child, that society should respect family integrity, and that we should allow those who will bear the burden of the consequences of the decision to have the major role in making the choice. However, respect for the authority of parent to make decisions for their child does not carry the same weight as the right of competent adults to make autonomous choices for themselves. There are limits to parental discretion in decision-making for their child and we will explore these limits more specifically in future chapters.

The ethical obligations of clinicians to a pregnant woman, a fetus, and a newborn are complex and evolve with the changing moral status of the fetus and newborn. It is not surprising that well-meaning clinicians may disagree about their ethical duties to a pregnant woman and her fetus. And it is not surprising that obstetricians and neonatologists have differing views of their obligations to a sick fetus who will become a neonate. These conflicting views are a clear demonstration of how moral obligations are not abstract concepts but are linked to professional roles and responsibilities.

In 1985, with the collaboration of an academic lawyer-ethicist, we initiated a teaching program at the medical center called Perinatal Law and Ethics Rounds. These monthly rounds were integrated into the regular perinatal teaching program of the departments of obstetrics and gynecology and pediatrics. These case-based discussions, which continue regularly to this day, directly address the complex legal and ethical relationships between a pregnant woman, her fetus, and her caregivers. Analysis of these cases enabled me to formulate and shape views on the concept of the fetus as a patient who warrants our respect and concern, and the unique role of the pregnant woman in making decisions that directly affect herself and her fetus. Some representative cases will enable us to explore some of the ethical issues that can occur in the process of giving birth to a baby.

TERM DELIVERY

Mary Brightman, the patient in Case 1, is a busy attorney who develops a birth plan at 36-weeks gestation in order to ensure that her personal preferences for the components of a good birth are respected when she goes into labor. For many competent and well-organized patients, the development of a birth plan is a useful way of controlling anxiety about the unfamiliar and chaotic circumstances of labor and delivery. This contemporary approach to asserting the views and values of a pregnant woman concerning how she wishes to be treated in labor is the response to decades of over medicalization of childbirth promulgated by obstetricians. Historically, well-intentioned clinicians, focused on the many things that might go wrong in labor that require immediate intervention, insisted that women in labor have an intravenous in place to administer medications if needed, a fetal monitor attached to continuously assess fetal well being, and the use of epidural anesthesia or drugs to reduce and control pain. Modern obstetric care is far more responsive to the desires and preferences of women in labor; and far more respectful of the birth process as a uniquely important life event that results in the creation of a new member of a family. Fifty years ago, almost all obstetricians were men; today, the vast majority of new obstetricians are women. This has been extraordinarily beneficial in helping the field of obstetrics to be more thoughtful and empathic to their patients.

Women have also changed in willingness to identify and assert their preferences. This creates a challenging and sometimes conflictual atmosphere during prenatal care and in the labor room as patients and clinicians negotiate and sometimes need to mediate value differences. Although most obstetricians are sensitive to their patient's wish to experience childbirth as a normal and natural life event, they are also aware that less than one hundred years ago many women died in childbirth and many fetuses were stillborn or severely damaged at delivery. It is the responsibility of obstetric professionals to prevent such tragic outcomes whenever possible, and they feel strongly about their ethical duties to both the woman and the fetus to carefully assess the progress of labor and intervene when needed. It is very hard to practice obstetrics. These clinicians must find the right balance between over medicalizing a normal pregnancy on the one hand, and, on the other hand, permitting a situation in which they are unaware of events that could negatively affect a woman and her fetus in labor.

Obstetricians need to encourage their patients to express their preferences. While acknowledging the patient's values and respecting their autonomy, clinicians need to create an atmosphere of shared decision-making about how best to proceed with labor and delivery. Clinicians need to remember that giving birth is a unique and awesome experience, and being invited to participate in this process is a privilege that should be cherished. Clinicians should assist patients in the creation of birth plans that express their values and preferences, but they must help their patients accept the possibility that medical events might require modifications of the original plan. This approach is helpful and sensitive, but additionally, it may alleviate a patient's guilt or disappointment if medical circumstances dictate greater intervention in labor and delivery than they anticipated. Physicians, as moral agents and professionals, must set some limits on their willingness to comply with patient requests. Women have the right to refuse medication, monitors, and epidurals. And women generally have the right to choose physicians whose values are similar to their own. But physicians also have the right to establish reasonable standards to determine which patients they will accept and which requests they will honor.

The birth plan that Mary Brightman developed was never discussed with her obstetrician. Instead, at the 37-week visit, Mary requested a scheduled cesarean delivery as soon as possible, so that she could return to work soon after the birth of her baby. Mary learned from her reading that preterm birth was risky for a baby, but that 37 weeks is the threshold for a term birth and, therefore, a low risk of problems. She also chose to control the route of the delivery realizing that induction of labor is often unsuccessful at 37 weeks and may result in a cesarean delivery after a difficult and debilitating attempt at labor. Mary was confident that her decision was sound and in the interests of her baby and her career. The baby would be born healthy and she would recover quickly from the surgery and be available to assist her client with some very important legal work. Mary's obstetrician was troubled by her request.

The use of term to describe all deliveries that occur after 37-weeks gestation suggests that these infants are all biologically mature and developmentally distinct from preterm infants who are born before 37 weeks. We now know this is neither factually accurate nor scientifically supportable. Historically, the designation of term beginning at 37-weeks gestation was determined somewhat arbitrarily to differentiate this period from the complications associated with earlier birth. Gestational age is a biologic continuum, and recent epidemiologic studies reveal that babies born at 37- and 38-weeks gestation have increased mortality and neonatal and long-term morbidity when compared with those born at 39 and 40 weeks. Although the overall risk of infant death from 37–41 weeks of pregnancy is low, the neonatal mortality rate is 50% higher for babies born at 37 weeks than those born at 40 weeks.

Elective cesarean delivery adds significant risk to the woman and the baby. The total cesarean-section rate including primary and repeat operative deliveries in the United Stats has increased dramatically over the past two decades and now accounts for over 30% of all births. When compared to vaginal birth, cesarean delivery is associated with substantially increased morbidity and even mortality for the woman, and increased respiratory morbidity for the baby. The American College of Obstetricians and Gynecologists strongly discourages elective cesarean delivery that is based solely on maternal request, and also discourages any elective delivery before 39 weeks of gestation. Over the last few years, great strides have been made in the area of obstetric quality improvement, resulting in a decrease in all elective deliveries before 39 weeks and the near elimination of cesarean deliveries solely on maternal request. This is an example of the successful prioritization of beneficence-based obligations to both mother and baby over respect for the autonomy of the mother. It is important to remember that autonomy is a negative right, it empowers capacitated adults with the right to refuse any medical treatment, but it does not give the adult patient the right to demand a treatment that the doctor does not accept as in their interests. Ms. Brightman's obstetrician explained all these facts to Mary and refused to deliver her at 37 weeks. The obstetrician agreed to induce labor at 39 weeks and hoped that a cesarean delivery would not be required.

The case of Tanya Chambers (Case 2) stands in stark contrast to the first case. Tanya refused to consent to a cesarean delivery when faced with a serious medical problem that jeopardized her life and that of her fetus. The clinicians caring for Ms. Chambers were greatly troubled by this situation. Their first response was to consider administering sedation to the patient through the indwelling intravenous in her arm so that they could take her to the operating room and perform a cesarean delivery without consent. Cooler heads prevailed, and remembering their duty to respect the autonomy of adult patients with the capacity to make healthcare decisions for themselves, they questioned whether Tanya's capacity to make decisions might be impaired. A psychiatrist was called for emergency consultation to assist in the assessment of capacity. If the psychiatrist determined that the patient lacked the capacity to understand the serious nature of her medical condition and was unable to make healthcare decisions for herself, the obstetricians could proceed with the emergent surgery without consent.

The psychiatric consultant hoped that he would find that Ms. Chambers demonstrated impaired capacity to make healthcare decisions for herself, because he wanted to enable the doctors to perform surgery in order to save her life and the life of the fetus. He was disappointed to find that she clearly had the capacity to make healthcare decisions; she understood her medical condition, the risks to herself and her fetus, and the potential consequences of refusal of the surgery. He recommended that the hospital urgently seek court involvement to allow the obstetricians to perform nonconsensual surgery.

There have been many legal cases requesting authorization of nonconsensual surgery on a pregnant woman to protect the interests of an otherwise viable fetus. Courts in the past have provided contradictory decisions in such cases. One court authorized nonconsensual surgery noting that the severe nature of the potential harm to the fetus warranted imposing the relatively low risk of surgery on the woman who was refusing cesarean delivery. Another court simply refused to authorize the surgery, holding that an adult who is competent to make the decision has a right to refuse treatment despite the potentially tragic consequences to herself or her fetus. Courts that have supported nonconsensual surgical delivery to save the life of a fetus have justified their decisions either by reference to the 1973 United States Supreme Court abortion decision, Roe v. Wade that held that after the fetus is viable, the state can prohibit abortion, or by relying on state child abuse and neglect statutes analogizing court ordered surgery for the survival of a viable fetus to court ordered treatment of a medically neglected child.

At first glance, the legal analysis by courts to justify nonconsensual surgery on pregnant women by reference to the abortion decision or the child-neglect statutes seems compelling, particularly from the perspective of anyone who wishes to protect the interests of the child who will be born. However, on more careful ethical examination of the issue, prioritizing the interests of the unborn child over its mother's fundamental right to refuse invasion of her body is troubling. The analysis by the courts seems flawed. The fact that the law has an interest in preventing certain consequences, the destruction of a viable fetus, does not mean that any and all action to prevent such consequences is warranted. There is a great difference between prohibiting active destruction of a viable fetus and requiring surgery on a competent adult to prevent potential harm to a fetus. The analogy to child neglect is also problematic. Although parents have clear legal duties to their children and may not refuse medically effective treatments for a child who will be imminently and irreversibly harmed by the refusal, women have not heretofore been held to have legally enforceable duties to place themselves at the considerable risk of surgery for the interests of their fetus or even for the interests of an already born child.

I would recommend against seeking court involvement in an attempt to override a capacitated patient's refusal of a recommended cesarean delivery. The act of seeking a court order may help the physician and the hospital feel better about this tragic situation by transferring to another entity the responsibility for the final decision; but court proceedings are adversarial and place the woman in a very difficult and inherently unfair position. She is unlikely to be able to adequately represent her interests while actively in labor, and because of the dramatic nature of the case and the urgent need for a decision, it is likely the court will move to preserve the fetus's life and override the competent refusal of the woman. Reversal of the court order on appeal many months later may provide a victory for the lawyer who argues the case and reveals the flaws in the court decision, but it does not undue the ethical wrong of invading the privacy and bodily integrity of the woman. Some would applaud the court for overriding the pregnant woman's choice and preventing the irreversible decision that will result in the death of the fetus. Although this view is understandable and may save the life of a future child, it can only be implemented by ignoring the universally held belief that respect for the autonomy of a capacitated adult should permit refusal of unwanted treatment.

PRETERM DELIVERY

Preterm birth, delivery before 37 completed weeks of gestation, is the leading cause of infant morbidity and mortality in the United States. It is a common and complex disorder with multiple causes. Each year, about 450,000, or close to 12%, (1 in 8) of all babies in the United States are born preterm. Because prematurity spans a wide range of gestational ages from the threshold of viability to the threshold of term birth, it can be divided into several categories: 22–26 weeks, profound preterm; 26–32 weeks, very preterm; 32–34 weeks, moderate preterm; and 34–37 weeks, late preterm. Between 1990 and 2006, there was more than a 20% increase in the rate of prematurity. Since that time, the rate of prematurity has leveled off and has recently begun to decrease. Advances in research and improvements in clinical care have resulted in survival for the vast majority of these tiny infants. Many of them thrive with minimal or no long-term problems, but a sizeable number are at risk for significant cognitive and neurodevelopmental problems. The economic cost of prematurity is astonishing; it is estimated that over 26 billion dollars per year is spent on the care of preterm infants in the United States.

The Threshold of Viability

Perhaps the most ethically troubling of all preterm infants are those at the threshold of viability, between 22 and 26 weeks gestation. Making decisions about labor, delivery, and resuscitation for fetuses in this group is a complex and difficult process for clinicians and families. United States studies reveal that survival rate to hospital discharge for infants born at 22-weeks gestation, the threshold of survivability, is about 5%. At 23-, 24-, and 25-weeks gestation, survival rates rise serially to about 30%, 60%, and 70%. Infants born at 23–25-weeks gestation who survive will frequently be affected by severe neurodevelopmental impairment. Moderate to severe cognitive impairment occurs in about 35–45% of the surviving children, and moderate to severe neuromotor impairment or cerebral palsy in 10–15%. Overall disability rates from mild to severe range from 75–90%. These are the kinds of data available to obstetricians and families when a pregnant woman at the threshold of viability shows signs of labor or becomes ill with hypertension that might jeopardize her health and the health of her fetus, or when a very preterm fetus shows signs of significant distress in utero. At these times, neonatologists are often consulted to share their experiences with similar cases, and outcome data from their specific unit. Although statistical probabilities are important to help frame the discussion, the outcome of an individual child is profoundly uncertain and impossible to predict.

Some obstetricians, aware of the risks of surgical delivery to the pregnant woman, are reluctant to recommend a cesarean section at 22- or 23-weeks gestation when a fetus shows signs of distress, believing it is unlikely that the fetus will survive. Others might view an emergency cesarean delivery as the only way to optimize the chance for fetal survival and the only way to increase the likelihood of a good outcome. Some women wish to take the risk associated with the surgery in order to increase the likelihood of survival of the infant regardless of the risk of poor outcome; others do not consent to surgery and would allow the fetus to die rather than risk the significant chance of a child surviving with severe neurodevelopmental morbidity. What degree of risk for a poor future quality of life for the child warrants the withholding of interventions to enhance the likelihood of survival?

Although data can be helpful, all these decisions are made in a unique context. The woman who is deciding about a possible cesarean delivery at 23-weeks gestation may be 38 years old and pregnant for the first time as a result of the fifth cycle of IVF; or she may be 22 years old in her first pregnancy that has been completely normal up to today; or she may be 32 years old with four healthy children at home. A careful exploration of her views and values, her hopes and fears, and her perception of the risks and benefits of the proposed courses of action, is critical to the process of decision- making.

When I am involved in this type of case, I make every effort to get to know the patient and her partner in order to learn about their hopes, fears, and values. I explain how difficult it is to predict the outcome for any individual fetus. I like to explain that many couples when faced with this type of decision often consider that the baby will either survive and be well or die. In fact, it is most likely that if the baby survives it will have some significant problems—problems that can be addressed within a loving and nurturing family, but serious problems nonetheless. I also share my view that if they agree to a cesarean delivery and the fetus is born alive, there will be other opportunities to consider whether to withhold or withdraw treatments after we have examined the child, obtained some initial tests, and have started to develop increased certainty about the child's likely outcome and possible future quality of life. Decisions to allow a fetus or child to die are irreversible. But, in cases when the potential for survival of the fetus and good outcome for the child is marginal at best, we should never place undue pressure on the family to risk surgical delivery, unless they are thoroughly convinced this is the right decision for them and for their baby.

Late-Preterm Delivery

Late-preterm delivery takes place between 34- and 37-weeks gestation. For decades, it has been the fastest growing group of preterm infants. Current obstetric practice considers 34 weeks gestation as a maturational milestone in prematurity. This is because mortality and the incidence of severe respiratory disease, bowel perforation, brain hemorrhage, and long-term morbidity in infants born after 34 weeks is far less than in those born prior to 34 weeks. Over 30% of the babies born late preterm are the result of a medically induced labor or performance of a cesarean section. The assumption that late-preterm infants will do well, make a smooth transition to extrauterine life, and behave more like term infants than smaller preterm babies has resulted in obstetricians recommending early delivery during this period without clear medical indications, and often without a good understanding of the potential consequences of this decision.

What are the ethical concerns about the increase in late-preterm birth? A substantial number of late-preterm infants, born early without a good medical indication, develop serious problems postdelivery. Several large studies have shown that obstetricians are inducing labor for maternal diabetes, hypertension, twins, and other complications of pregnancy at gestational ages earlier than medically indicated ostensibly to prevent the need for an emergency delivery and to decrease the risk of birth asphyxia but without evidence of the necessity to intervene at that early a gestational age. And, like Mary Brightman in Case 1, many women are seeking early delivery for various personal reasons. In addition, many obstetricians have been scheduling inductions and repeat cesarean deliveries for their own convenience. It is important to realize that if the gestational age of the pregnancy is based solely on maternal history with no confirmatory ultrasound examination performed in the first weeks of pregnancy, gestational dating at 37 or 38 weeks can be off by as much as two weeks, resulting in the birth of a late-preterm infant even if delivery is anticipated at 37 or 38 weeks.

Greater awareness of the complications of late-preterm birth, combined with a major educational and quality improvement campaign for obstetricians and a public education campaign for pregnant women, has made the problem of late-preterm delivery a national public-health priority. Efforts in recent years have significantly decreased the number of nonmedically indicated preterm births, and have decreased the overall incidence of prematurity in the United States. Ensuring that obstetricians and pregnant women are knowledgeable about the risks of early delivery, and decreasing the requests and recommendations for early induction or cesarean delivery can result in decreasing mortality and morbidity among neonates. Prioritizing beneficence-based ethical obligations to late-preterm and early-term infants, and transforming the practice of obstetrics in America to decrease inductions and surgical deliveries before 39 weeks gestation, has significantly decreased neonatal morbidity and mortality.

DO-NOT-RESUSCITATE ORDERS IN THE DELIVERY ROOM

Advance directives concerning resuscitation and intubation are increasingly common in medical care. Orders not to attempt resuscitation (DNR), written by physicians in response to the wishes of capacitated patients or their surrogates, are used to ensure that patients' autonomous wishes and their interest in precluding the prolongation of suffering or dying are respected. DNR orders obligate physicians to make no efforts to revive a patient who has suffered a cardiovascular arrest. In the case of infants, parents and guardians are generally given the authority as surrogates to make these decisions. There is an increasing desire to use DNR orders in the delivery room. This phenomenon is the result of enhanced capability by obstetricians to accurately assess gestational age and diagnose fetal abnormalities in utero. Also, obstetricians voice the concern that some neonatologists are unwilling to withhold resuscitative efforts from any live-born baby regardless of gestational age or degree of abnormality. Well-intentioned obstetricians have used antenatal DNR orders to document parents' wishes to refuse technological interventions to prolong the life of their child after birth. Are DNR orders the appropriate way to express parents' wishes? What should be done about resuscitation in the case of the birth of a baby at the threshold of viability, or a more developed fetus with a severe congenital abnormality, when parents request that "nothing be done" to prolong the life of a baby about to be born?

Although I believe it is sometimes appropriate to withhold resuscitative efforts from a newborn immediately after birth, I do not think that DNR orders and other antenatal advance directives that preclude resuscitation are the appropriate way to deal with these concerns. Resuscitative efforts in a delivery room are quite different from the circumstances generally associated with providing cardiopulmonary resuscitation to a patient who has a sudden cessation of heart function or is in the process of dying due to a serious or chronic illness. Fetal transition from intrauterine to extra-uterine life is generally associated with a good heart rate immediately after birth and a strong biologic drive on the part of the newborn to initiate breathing. In term infants, clearing the airway with mild suctioning, and stimulating a baby are usually the only resuscitative efforts required. It is difficult to predict before birth which resuscitative measures, if any, will be needed for a specific patient. In fact, many babies will survive without any assistance after birth. Should a DNR order result in the withholding of simple noninvasive support such as clearing the airway and oxygen administered by mask? Withholding basic measures, short of intubation and cardiovascular resuscitation, may result in a poorer outcome but not in the death of the newborn.

Prenatal DNR orders are neither necessary nor sufficient to determine the actions of clinicians responsible for delivery-room resuscitations. Neonatologists have an obligation to each newborn to assess the patient, confirm the gestational age, diagnosis, suspected abnormal findings, and determine the level of resuscitative effort that is appropriate for that patient. A prenatal DNR order should not be necessary to ensure a family's wishes not to prolong their child's suffering after birth. The absence of a DNR order does not create new obligations on the part of the clinician caring for a newborn to provide treatments that are not in the best interests of the infant and that will only prolong suffering. And a prenatal DNR order is not sufficient to preclude the attendance of a neonatologist or other clinician skilled in resuscitation at a delivery, nor is it sufficient to limit a doctor's actions in response to an infant who appears to be reasonably healthy and responsive.

Resuscitative efforts should be tailored to the needs and interests of each patient, taking into consideration the wishes and values of the parents. Antenatal consultation with parents to clarify their views and values is critical. Clinicians are obligated to assess the newborn and provide only those treatments deemed to be in the interests of the patient. Knowing the family's wishes should impact on the clinician's decisions about the appropriate level and duration of resuscitative efforts, but the family's wishes should not be determinative of the clinician's action in all cases.

It is often helpful when communicating with families prenatally, to reassure them that the initiation of treatment does not obligate continuation. Withdrawal of technological support and allowing the child to die after a thorough assessment is often a better option to ensure the parents wishes are fulfilled while respecting the interests of the neonate. We will discuss this in greater detail in the next chapter.

MATERNAL CATASTROPHE AND BRAIN DEATH

It is possible for a child to be born after its mother is in coma or dead. Massive intracranial hemorrhage from arterial aneurysm, automobile accidents, gunshot wounds and other catastrophic events may significantly jeopardize the life and health of a pregnant woman and her fetus. The survival and future outcome for both are dependent on several factors including: the underlying cause and severity of the injury, whether the patient is observed at the time of the injury, the rapidity and effectiveness of the resuscitative efforts, and the time to arrival at a hospital. When a pregnant woman arrives in a hospital emergency department after a catastrophic injury, there are urgent clinical and ethical concerns. Resuscitation of the woman is critical, but simultaneous delivery of the fetus may be the only hope for fetal survival.

Emergency medicine physicians, in collaboration with obstetricians, must make rapid assessments about the gestational age and immediate well-being of the fetus. If the fetus appears to be viable and in reasonable condition, an emergency cesarean delivery may be indicated, as long as it does not jeopardize efforts to revive and stabilize the woman. All resuscitative efforts for the woman should be continued until a decision is made about the fetus. There is always concern about the effect of maternal hypotension and lack of uterine perfusion on the fetus. The fetal heart may be beating at a normal rate, but its brain may be severely compromised. If other family members are available in the emergency department, it may be helpful to elicit their thoughts about what the woman might have wanted in this situation and about the family's views about efforts to save the fetus. There are many reports of babies born by immediate cesarean delivery in these circumstances who do well clinically.

I have cared for several term newborns born by postmortem cesarean section in the emergency department, after the cardiac arrest of their mothers. Each was severely neurologically damaged. I have supported the father and other family members who have had to cope with both the loss of their loved one and the birth of a child with severe neurologic abnormalities. I must disclose that I am biased against postmortem cesarean delivery under these circumstances, unless the mother's cardiac rate, rhythm, and blood pressure can be brought back to normal within a very few minutes of the initial event. We know that 5–10 minutes of poor perfusion to the fetal brain will have devastating results and that arrival at the emergency department often takes longer than that. Resuscitative efforts, including ventilation and fluid replacement in the field and on the way to the hospital, are critical in determining the outcome for the baby. Detailed knowledge of what has transpired should be part of the decision-making process about whether there should be an attempt to save the fetus.

Sometimes resuscitative efforts can result in immediate cardiovascular stabilization of the pregnant woman, resulting in a stable fetus as well. In this situation, an immediate cesarean delivery is not needed and further stabilization of the woman and fetus is possible. Critical care of the woman, including neurosurgery, trauma surgery, or other stabilizing procedures can be accomplished with continual monitoring of fetal well-being. It may be determined that the woman is severely neurologically damaged or even brain dead but that the fetus is stable. The diagnosis of brain death in the pregnant woman may require several hours or days. During this time, every effort should be made to assess fetal gestational age and well-being. Discussions should ensue with the father of the fetus and other family members about the possibility of continuing the pregnancy, even if the mother is neurologically impaired or brain dead.

Many states in the United States will not respect the prior wishes of a critically and terminally ill pregnant woman who has lost the capacity to make decisions for herself to withdraw life support, and they will not permit family members to act as surrogates to make the decision that will allow the woman and fetus to die. These states insist on maintaining life support in the interests of the fetus. Some of these laws require that life support measures continue whatever the gestational age and no matter whether the fetus is considered viable. I believe this is a grave mistake and blatantly unjust. Ignoring the wishes of a formerly capacitated adult and her surrogates is not appropriate. Prioritizing the interests of a previable fetus that may be severely impaired, and forcing a family to accept the risk of having to care for a child who may be severely disabled is contemptuous of individual rights, mean spirited, and unreasonable. In this pluralistic society, one that is very diverse and not a theocracy, it seems to me that imposing such laws, based primarily on religious beliefs, is just wrong.

One state has interpreted its law to argue that even a woman declared brain dead must be maintained with technological support to sustain the fetus to viability regardless of the wishes of her family. The woman, at the end of the first trimester of pregnancy, became brain dead after cardiac arrest at home from a pulmonary embolus. The state authorities chose to disregard the prior wishes of the woman and the beliefs of her surrogates, prioritizing the putative interests of the fetus, and forcing the woman to be maintained on machines to support the physiologic functions of her body after death. Some commentators have argued that since the pregnant woman is dead, she has no interests, her surrogates have no authority to make decisions for her concerning the fetus, and clinicians have no ethical obligations to her. I find this line of reasoning very troubling. Respect for a former patient, her wishes concerning the circumstances of her death, and the disposition of her body should have meaning to clinicians and to the state. Physicians are not permitted to practice procedures on dead bodies without explicit prior permission, and clinicians are expected to respect the dead body and permit family members to prepare for its burial or cremation consistent with their religious or secular beliefs. Even when deceased patients have no relatives or friends to claim the body, the hospital treats the body with respect and arranges for a publicly funded burial.

Maintaining a brain-dead body in a stable physiologic state that can support a developing fetus is very difficult and risky for the fetus. Brain-dead bodies develop extremes of cardiovascular instability, temperature-control problems, panhypopituitarism with consequent multiple endocrine disorders, and autonomic nervous system instability. Even in the best of clinical circumstances, it is impossible to predict the outcome of a fetus after long-term support in its brain-dead mother.

Nevertheless, some families do request that their deceased loved one's body be supported to allow a fetus to develop to viability. There are about 30 such cases reported in the medical literature, but it is likely that there are many more cases that have actually occurred. Several years ago, at the request of a father and grandparents, I had the opportunity to assist in the care of a brain-dead pregnant woman and to assist at the birth of their baby. The mother had suffered a brain hemorrhage from a cerebral aneurysm at 22 weeks of pregnancy. She arrived in the emergency department conscious with a good blood pressure. Her condition deteriorated in the hospital and, despite emergent neurosurgery in an attempt to save her life, she became brain dead. During all these efforts, the doctors were able to maintain physiologic stability of the woman's vital signs and the fetus appeared to remain stable under constant monitoring. The family asked us to try to save the baby. They saw this effort as allowing some good to come from the tragic death of their loved one. The father spoke of the child as his wife's legacy and a reincarnation of her spirit. He mourned his wife's death each day, as we helped the fetus grow and develop inside the body of its mother that had become its incubator. Several weeks later, at about 27-weeks gestation, we were no longer able to stabilize the physiologic environment of the brain-dead body and could not maintain stable uterine blood flow needed for fetal well-being. A two-pound baby boy was delivered by cesarean section. He did well in the neonatal intensive care unit and was discharged home to a loving family with a very good prognosis.

I respected this family's decision and was happy to be able to participate in the care. Nonetheless, I believe it would have been ethically acceptable for the family to have chosen a different path, one that accepted the brain death of their loved one as the end of her life and of the pregnancy.

BEHAVIORS DURING PREGNANCY THAT JEOPARDIZE THE FETUS

I have argued in this chapter that a pregnant woman has beneficence-based ethical obligations to behave in a manner that maintains her health and the health of her fetus if she has decided the fetus will become a child. What should clinicians do about patients who exhibit behaviors during pregnancy that jeopardize the health of the fetus, such as smoking, drinking alcohol, taking illicit drugs, or abusing prescription drugs? Smoking, use of alcohol, and drug abuse during pregnancy occur across all cultural and socioeconomic lines, but the greatest impact appears to be among economically disadvantaged and medically underserved minority groups. Surveys of women of child-bearing age reveal that as many as 60% drink alcohol and 30% have used an illegal drug in the year preceding the pregnancy. Studies of urine samples from pregnant women report that 5–15% have used an illicit substance within the month prior to delivery. Despite similar rates of substance abuse among African-American and white women in one study, black women were ten times more likely than white women to be reported to state child-welfare authorities, and poor women were more likely to be reported regardless of race.

Clinicians caring for women who are not pregnant clearly have beneficence-based duties to help each patient to change her health-risking behaviors. A patient's refusal to change a harmful behavior, while potentially damaging to her well-being, does not rise to the level of justifying interference with her liberty in any way beyond repeated attempts at counseling, education, and persuasion. However, when that patient becomes pregnant and her behavior risks the health and well-being of her fetus, many argue that there is adequate justification to interfere with her liberty for the sake of her future baby. This view has resulted in laws in several states that obligate clinicians to question pregnant women about illicit substance use and to test urine samples for signs of drug use during pregnancy. Clinicians become fetal police, required to make reports of substance use to child-welfare authorities, rather than referring women to social-service agencies for psychological and substance abuse counseling. State child-welfare agencies have incarcerated pregnant women in an attempt to prevent the transfer of potentially harmful substances to fetuses. This punitive approach to substance abuse during pregnancy ignores the fact that these chemicals may be physically or psychologically addictive resulting in the woman not being able to stop their use without help. And the penal system generally has few social or psychological services available to help the women with this problem.

Legal scholars justify these laws by reference to provisions of the Supreme Court abortion decision and state child-abuse laws in a manner similar to the justification of forced cesarean deliveries discussed earlier in this chapter. I think it is even harder to justify incarcerating a pregnant woman for substance use than it is to impose nonconsensual surgery when her fetus is in acute distress. The affects on the fetus of substances of abuse vary widely, and it is very hard to predict whether an individual fetus will be harmed. Also, incarceration of a pregnant woman has never been shown to have a long-term positive impact on a future child. Perhaps most importantly, the threat of state intervention and possible incarceration during pregnancy has not been shown to be a deterrent to substance abuse, but has been shown to cause women to flee the healthcare system resulting in the potential for far greater harm to themselves and their future children. It seems foolish to place these medical and social problems in the realm of the criminal justice system. Incarcerating women and ignoring the potential for medical and behavioral intervention to assist pregnant women to deal with a substance-abuse problem, results in far more negative consequences than positive outcomes. States should prioritize social interventions to prevent, treat, and ameliorate substance use rather than use punitive approaches to punish addictive behavior.

FINAL THOUGHTS

The ethical obligations of a clinician to a pregnant woman and her fetus are complex and evolve during the course of gestation. Although obstetricians clearly have ethical obligations to a pregnant woman to act in a way that promotes her health-related interests and respects her views and values, they also have beneficence-based duties to the fetus who is intended to become a child. These duties to the fetus need not be based on the moral status of the fetus but, rather, on the relationship of the physician to the fetus as a patient. It is not surprising that this unique circumstance, a clinician simultaneously treating two patients with possibly conflicting interests, is difficult to manage even for the most capable obstetricians.

Each pregnant woman has beneficence-based obligations to their fetus who will become a child. These duties are not unlimited and do not require the woman to place herself at undue risk for the benefit of the future child. I have avoided the language of "maternal–fetal conflict" to describe those instances when the values of a woman do not prioritize the outcome of her fetus over her assessment of her own best interest. I believe that invoking the language of *conflict* pits one party against the other and is less likely to result in maximizing benefits to both.

Respect for both patients, the woman and the fetus, requires that clinicians weigh all the consequences of proposed treatments to both parties, make recommendations that appear to maximize benefits to both, and use moral persuasion when necessary to convince women to take reasonable risks to optimize fetal outcomes. But clinicians should not let their concern for one party denigrate their respect for the other. Recommendations must take into account the woman's values and preferences, and when physicians and women disagree about what is best, the woman's choice should prevail. When pregnant women are respected and do not fear that their views and values are being ignored or trivialized, they are far more likely to make those choices that optimize outcomes for all concerned.

ADDITIONAL READINGS

Campbell DE, Fleischman AR. Limits of viability: dilemmas, decisions and decision makers. *Am J Perinat,* 2001; 18:117–128.

Esmaeilzadeh M, Dictus C, Kayvanpour E, Sedaghat-Hamedani F, et al. One life ends, another begins: Management of a brain dead pregnant mother—A systematic review. *BMC Med,* 2010; 8:74.

Fleischman AR, Chervenak FA, McCullough LB. The physicians moral obligations to the pregnant woman, the fetus, and the child. *Sem Perinat,* 1998; 22(3): 184–188.

Fleischman AR, Oinuma M, Clark SL. Rethinking the definition of "term pregnancy." *Obstet & Gyn* 2010; 116(1): 136–139.

Fleischman AR, Rhoden NK. Perinatal law and ethics rounds. *Obstet & Gyn,* 1988; 71(5): 790–795.

Mohan SS, Jain L. Late preterm birth: preventable prematurity? *Clin Perinat,* 2011; 38 (3): 547–555.

Yellin PB, Fleischman AR: DNR in the DR? *J Perinatol,* 1995; 15:232–236.

CHAPTER 4

Ethical Issues in Neonatal Intensive Care

Case 1

Monica Madison is a 26-year-old neurosurgical intensive care nurse who had a "perfect" pregnancy until at 24.5 weeks gestation (15 weeks early) she experienced a gush of fluid that wet her slacks, indicating preterm premature rupture of the membranes that surround her fetus. She called her husband, Dr. Jason Madison, a 29-year-old resident in orthopedics, and proceeded to her obstetrician's office. Monica was examined, assessed and admitted to the hospital labor and delivery area for observation. Over the ensuing six hours, labor commenced and could not be stopped with tocolytic agents. Jason and Monica were devastated. They knew that the chance for survival of their baby was small and if the baby survived it was likely to have serious neurologic problems.

Their son, Joey, was born and stabilized in the delivery room. Joey weighed 610 grams (about 1 pound 4 ounces). Dr. Madison followed the neonatal team to the intensive care unit where they placed Joey on a respirator, inserted arterial and venous lines, and provided a dose of "surfactant" directly into the trachea in an attempt to decrease the severity of the lung disease that is present in very preterm infants. The attending neonatologist, Dr. Kaufman, explained to Dr. Madison that Joey was stable, active, and responding to treatment; he hoped for a good outcome. Dr. Madison asked Dr. Kaufman about the possibility that Joey would survive but suffer a life with disabilities. Dr. Kaufman remained optimistic, sharing many stories about 24-week infants who did well.

During that night Joey had a turn for the worse. He ceased being active, needed a small blood transfusion, received medication to support his blood pressure, and required increased respirator settings to maintain ventilation and oxygenation. When Monica Mason visited Joey's bedside early in the morning, she was informed by the nurse that the ultrasound technician said that there appeared to be substantial bleeding inside the ventricles in Joey's brain. For Jason and Monica, this was confirmation that Joey would not do well. They decided to ask Dr. Kaufman to withdraw the technology and to allow Monica to hold Joey as he died. Dr. Kaufman refused their request. He argued that continued treatment was in Joey's best interests and that he had an obligation to continue to support Joey. He described other children he had cared for who were thriving despite this type of brain injury in the first days of life.

Case 2

Carmen Rodriquez is a 28-year-old woman in her second pregnancy at 39 weeks gestation. The pregnancy went very well with no problems until a few hours before she arrived at the hospital accompanied by her husband Ramon, complaining that "her fetus is not moving." After a rapid evaluation, it became clear that the fetal heart beat was slow and irregular. The doctors explained to Mr. and Mrs. Rodriquez that an emergency cesarean section was needed. Carmen agreed to the surgery and was whisked back to the operating room for immediate delivery. Less than 15 minutes from the time the Rodriquez's arrived at the hospital, their baby boy, Juan, was born. He was pale, blue, and not moving with a very slow heart rate of 60 beats per minute. Resuscitative efforts began immediately with intubation for ventilatory support, cardiac compressions to generate some perfusion, and the insertion of an umbilical line for fluids and medications. Juan was severely acidotic at birth but responded to the resuscitation with an increase of his heart rate and blood pressure to normal. He was rapidly stabilized and transferred to the neonatal intensive care unit.

In the NICU, Juan was pink and perfusing well with normal vital signs and good oxygenation, but he did not move at all except for what appeared to be localized seizure activity on his right side. The doctors explained to Mr. and Mrs. Rodriquez that Juan was extremely ill and that his brain had sustained a very serious insult. Carmen and Ramon cried at the bedside and prayed to God to help their son. They asked the doctors and nurses why this happened and what did they do wrong? The doctors explained that they were not sure why this occurred, it might have been a compression of the umbilical cord in utero; but whatever the cause, it was not predictable or preventable.

After several days of aggressive treatment to decrease brain swelling, control the seizures, and maintain metabolic homeostasis, Juan was still having no spontaneous movement. His EEG and MRI studies revealed severe brain damage from lack of oxygen. Neurology consultants predicted a dismal outcome for Juan. The doctors met with Carmen and Ramon on day six of life to discuss the possibility of withdrawing the respirator and allowing Juan to die. The Rodriquez's were thankful for all the efforts the clinicians had done to help their son. They were angry at God for not intervening on Juan's behalf, but they could not agree to withdraw treatment and allow Juan to die. They hoped for a miracle and asked the doctors and nurses to continue to "do everything they could" to save their son.

The sickest patients in academic medical centers are frequently also the smallest. They reside in neonatal intensive care units, suffering from the serious consequences of preterm birth, congenital abnormalities, chronic and acute infections, and perinatal asphyxia (lack of oxygen affecting the brain and other organs). About 10% of the four million babies born each year in the United States require some level of intensive care. The modern neonatal intensive care unit provides both highly competent professionals and extraordinary technology that combine to save the lives of the vast majority of these sick patients. Saving the life of a sick infant is a very rewarding experience, but it can be associated with significant long-term consequences for the child and family. A great deal is at stake. Life, death, and disability are constantly on the minds of the clinicians and families who unite at the bedside of these vulnerable babies. Most parents have never seen or been inside a neonatal unit. They are first struck by the fact that their baby seems very vulnerable, cared for on an open bed; kept warm by heat provided overhead; and surrounded by monitors, ventilators, and other equipment. Neonatal intensive care units have all the same types of equipment that are available in an adult unit, but the small size of the neonatal patients make the equipment look larger and more foreboding.

The special care of premature and sick newborns is not new, it began in the United States in the early 1900s, focusing on maintaining temperature regulation and creating special techniques and formulas to feed these very vulnerable infants. Recognizing that babies weighing less than four pounds survived at a rate four times greater if their body temperatures could be maintained in the normal range, led to the design of the incubator. By the early 1920s, hospitals began to have special newborn baby units for the care of preterm and low birthweight infants. Artificial formulas were developed to replace breast milk for these sick and small infants, and over the following 25 years, research to determine requirements for fluid, protein, and calories enabled the creation of cow-milk based formulas specifically designed for sick term and preterm infants.

After World War II, when the country began to focus on healthcare delivery and preventive health, the field of pediatrics grew and the care of sick newborns in special care units became commonplace. In 1963, Patrick Bouvier Kennedy, the son of the president, was born preterm at 34.5-weeks gestation and weighed 4 pounds 10.5 ounces. He suffered from respiratory distress and despite aggressive treatment and transfer to a major academic medical center, he died on the third day of life. He was not placed on a respirator because none was available for newborns in that children's hospital.

During the 1960s, monitoring equipment and respirators that had been developed for adults suffering from heart attacks or used postoperatively were adapted for use in newborns in special care units. The development of miniaturized technology for use in human space travel accelerated the creation of smaller and more sophisticated equipment. The 1960s and 1970s saw the creation of neonatal intensive care units in every major hospital in the United States and the development of neonatology as a bona fide subspecialty of pediatrics.

A BRIEF HISTORY OF DECISION-MAKING
FOR CRITICALLY ILL NEONATES

As a medical student in the 1960s, I became interested in pediatrics and took a fourth-year elective subinternship in the neonatal intensive care unit. One night in 1969, when I was on call, I was sent to the delivery room for the impending vaginal birth of a two- pound (900 gram), 28-week gestation preterm infant. The baby looked good at birth but she was clearly having difficulty breathing. I dried and warmed her and administered oxygen. Breathing became more labored, so I placed a small endotracheal tube in the baby's windpipe and began to ventilate her with the help of an ambu bag connected to the tube. I called the neonatal intensive care unit and told the nursing staff that I was coming over from the delivery room with a new admission and to please set up a respirator. I had a brief conversation with the parents in the delivery room explaining that their daughter was a very small and very sick baby but we would try to do everything we could for her. They thanked me and watched as I pushed their little girl in a small transport incubator out of the room.

It was about 3 A.M. when I arrived in the unit. The nurses greeted me with skeptical looks and the head nurse calmly explained that babies of this size and gestational age were not placed on respirators because none had ever survived in this unit. The nurses suggested that I take the tube out of the baby's trachea, place her in oxygen, and hope that she would be able to survive without technological support. They recommended that I go counsel the family that we were doing everything we could, but the outlook was grave. I chose to not extubate the patient, but since they refused to provide a respirator for the baby, I had to sit by the incubator and ventilate the infant by hand with an ambu bag.

At 7 A.M. the director of the unit arrived. He had been informed by a phone call from the head nurse about what was happening in the unit. He asked one of the nurses to take the ambu bag from me and to continue to ventilate the patient while we went to his office to have a cup of coffee. The director explained to me that inflicting pain and suffering that prolonged an inevitable death was unethical. He had never had a baby survive in his unit at this birth weight and gestational age and, therefore, he could not let me continue to ventilate the baby.

We went back to the bedside of the baby where the unit director took out the endotracheal tube. The baby died within a few hours. This was my first personal exposure to a neonatal ethical dilemma. It seemed right not to cause pain or prolong suffering in a patient who would inevitably die, but this little girl seemed strong, and her family and I were clearly hoping that she would pull through. I learned that physicians play a critical role in deciding what treatments were medically indicated and would be provided to sick patients, and that in this instance parents' hopes did not play a role in these choices.

When the U.S. Supreme Court, in 1973, decided the case of Roe v. Wade to deal with the abortion dilemma, they defined viability as 28-weeks gestation. Twenty-eight weeks gestation was not the absolute biologic threshold of viability in 1973; about 10% of babies born at 28 weeks survived. But using 28 weeks as the boundary for the definition of viability was a reasonable decision in 1973. The Court held that after the fetus is viable, the state can prohibit abortion unless it is needed to protect the woman's life or health. The Court was seeking to balance the rights of a pregnant woman to determine what happens to her own body against the interests of the fetus after it is viable and could potentially survive outside the uterus with assistance.

In 1973, two physicians from Yale University School of Medicine published a landmark paper in the New England Journal of Medicine describing the process of withholding treatment from infants in order to allow them to die in the special care nursery. Although physicians were aware that similar decisions were being made in nurseries throughout the United States, this was the first public acknowledgment that clinicians and families were facing ethically complex decisions and allowing infants to die in neonatal intensive care units. The article reviewed neonatal deaths over a 30-month period, 14% of which were related to withholding or withdrawing treatment. In this group were infants with multiple congenital anomalies, central nervous system disorders, myelomeningocoele (spina bifida), short bowel syndrome, and genetic abnormalities including Down Syndrome. The authors described the process by which physicians and families in a collaborative decision concluded that the prognosis for meaningful life was extremely poor or hopeless and, therefore, rejected further treatment. They ably described and discussed all the issues relevant to decision-making for critically ill and disabled infants in neonatal intensive care units. They noted that these choices were often fraught with prognostic uncertainty and were agonizing for physicians and families, but they strongly urged that such choices should be left to parents with the guidance of physicians. They also concluded that the issue of withholding treatment from critically ill and disabled children had to be faced, since not deciding, insisting that treatment continue, is an arbitrary and potentially devastating default decision. I agreed with their wise analysis when I first read the article then, and I continue to share their view now.

In 1979, Congress created the President's Commission for the Study of Ethical Problems in Medicine and Biomedical and Behavioral Research. This group faced the issues concerning healthcare decisions for seriously ill neonates in one of its volumes published in 1983. They addressed the fact that parents are surrogate decision-makers for infants, making decisions for their children who cannot speak for themselves. The Commission argued that parents should seek to determine what is in the best interests of their child, taking into account quality-of-life indicators such as the child's amount of suffering and potential for relief, the expected duration of life, the severity of dysfunction, the potential for personal satisfaction and enjoyment of life, and the possibility of developing the capacity for self-determination. They concluded that parents and physicians should share the responsibility for making hard decisions for seriously ill neonates. When treatment is clearly beneficial, it should be provided regardless of whether or not parents agree, but for cases in which the benefits of treatment are ambiguous or uncertain, parents should have the authority to determine whether treatment is provided or foregone. When treatment is considered futile, cannot provide benefit, and may only prolong or increase suffering, life-extending treatment should not be provided, even if parents insist on it. The Commission went on to recommend that when the benefits of therapy are unclear, an ethics committee might be helpful to review the decision-making process. It specifically noted that decisional review might be most important when foregoing life-sustaining treatment was proposed because of a physical or mental handicap.

Although this learned Presidential Commission was grappling with making recommendations for decision-making for babies who are seriously ill, the executive branch of the federal government was faced with a crisis when asked to respond to the case of Baby Doe, a baby born in Bloomington, Indiana in April, 1982. Baby Doe was born with Down Syndrome, Trisomy 21, a genetic disorder in which there are three copies of the 21st chromosome instead of the normal two. Children with Down Syndrome have some characteristic facial features, some degree of cognitive impairment, and often have congenital anomalies of the heart or bowel. Baby Doe was born with a blockage in the esophagus and a fistula, or open connection, between his esophagus and trachea. Because of the obvious facial features of Down Syndrome, and the known association of that disorder with mental retardation, the physician caring for the family recommended that no surgery be performed to correct the esophageal blockage, and that the baby be allowed to die. The parents concurred with the recommendation. Caregivers inside the hospital sought court intervention to mandate surgery, but judges determined that it was within the authority of the parents to refuse to consent to surgery. Baby Doe died in the hospital after six days of life, presumably from dehydration.

President Reagan and U. S. Surgeon General Koop, a former pediatric surgeon who had operated on many children with Down Syndrome and bowel obstruction, reacted to this event by promulgating federal regulations mandating treatment for all neonates, precluding parents or physicians from withholding or withdrawing treatments from critically ill infants. They promulgated an executive order that mandated the posting of signs in delivery rooms and nurseries in every hospital asking people to call a hotline number if anyone observed discriminatory withholding of treatments from a neonate. The call would then potentially trigger an investigation by federal agents.

These draconian regulations were withdrawn after substantial protest from pediatric groups and family advocates, to be replaced by compromise legislation, the Child Abuse Prevention and Treatment Act Amendments of 1984. This act required each state to accept new rules in order to receive federal funding for their child abuse and medical neglect programs. The new Baby Doe Rules redefined *medical neglect* to include the discriminatory withholding of medically indicated treatment from a disabled infant with a life-threatening condition. The concept of medical neglect had been used previously by states to justify court intervention to override parental refusal of efficacious treatments when imminent and permanent harm might occur if the treatments were not provided. The Act stated that the determination of what counts as medically indicated or beneficial treatment for a sick neonate be left to the treating physician based on "reasonable medical judgment." The rules specify three instances in which the withholding of medical treatment is justified:

"(1) the infant is chronically and irreversibly comatose;
(2) the provision of such treatment would merely prolong dying, not be effective in ameliorating or correcting all of the infant's life threatening conditions; or otherwise be futile in terms of survival of the infant; or
(3) the provision of such treatment would be virtually futile in terms of the survival of the infant, and the treatment itself under such circumstances would be inhumane."

Many commentators severely criticized these new rules and feared that physicians treating neonates would no longer allow parents to withhold or withdraw treatments from critically and seriously ill children. In fact, some neonatologists and many hospital attorneys interpreted the rules narrowly. This resulted in aggressive treatment being imposed on neonates over the objection of their families. I believed that these regulations could be interpreted to permit collaborative decision-making among clinicians and parents that was unchanged from practices before the Baby Doe crisis. The Act permitted physicians to determine which treatments were medically indicated based on reasonable medical judgment; families were not precluded from being involved in decision-making; and, most importantly, the third provision of the act that allowed treatment to be withheld if it would be "virtually futile in terms of survival" permitted physicians to make that determination as well as to determine if the treatment in those circumstances would be "inhumane." This permitted decisions to be made consistent with all the quality-of-life indicators suggested by the Presidential Commission as long as the physician was willing to state that continued treatment was virtually futile in term of the infant's survival. We had many debates about what "virtually futile in terms of survival" meant, and concluded that the term was unclear; I concluded the likelihood of death was far less important than the potential for future suffering, the level of dysfunction, and the future quality of the child's life.

Another famous Baby Doe was born in 1983, a little girl, Jane Doe. She was born on Long Island, New York, with spina bifida, hydrocephalus (fluid filled ventricles inside the brain) and microcephaly (a small head). The physicians caring for Jane Doe offered her parents the option of "comfort care" rather than surgical intervention to close the defect in the lower spine and place a shunt in her head to drain the accumulating fluid into her abdomen. The parents accepted the fact that comfort measures would alleviate any pain or suffering, but would likely result in Jane's death in a few weeks to months. It is unclear how news of this case reached a well-known right-to-life attorney in Albany, New York, but he sought court intervention to force surgical treatment to save the baby's life. New York courts ruled that the family, in consultation with a licensed physician, had the authority to determine the appropriate treatment plan for their child. This case was appealed to the U.S. Supreme Court. In 1986, the Supreme Court ruled that the Baby Doe regulations were not applicable to this case because there was no discrimination, and that parents, in consultation with physicians, are the appropriate decision-makers for their critically and chronically ill children. This decision made most of the neonatal community comfortable with the approaches we had been using to engage families in making quality-of-life-based choices for their infants. The Child Abuse Amendment and its major focus on the potential for the patient's survival became less important in decision-making and was virtually ignored.

INFANT BIOETHICS COMMITTEES

The President's Commission and the American Academy of Pediatrics, in 1983, recommended that infant bioethics committees might be helpful when decisions are contemplated to withhold or withdraw life-sustaining treatment from a seriously ill neonate. We created such a committee encompassing the three large neonatal units in our program, outlined its membership, developed its operating principles, and defined its functions. We began to review cases in February of 1984. Our operating principles included the belief that each newborn possesses an intrinsic dignity and worth that entitles the infant to receive all forms of care and treatment thought to be in his or her best interests and conducive to his or her well-being. We argued that parents bear the principal moral responsibility and decision-making authority for their infant and should be the surrogates for the child unless they choose a course of action that is clearly against the infant's best interest. We also recognized that although medical treatments that are in the best interest of a patient should always be provided, whether a medical treatment is in the best interest of a particular infant is sometimes uncertain. We rejected unfettered vitalism, and embraced a quality-of-life perspective, although individual members disagreed on what might constitute a future quality of life that could justify a parent's decision to allow a child to die. However, we all agreed that the family should have the authority to make decisions about withholding or withdrawing of life-sustaining treatment in any case when that decision was not clearly against the child's interest. The committee provided review and consultation, but the family and the attending physician maintained the ultimate authority to make the clinical decisions that affected the child.

Much has been written about infant bioethics committees, and several controversial issues remain unresolved. Who should be permitted to request an ethics committee consultation? Should families be able to refuse an ethics consultation? And, should there be some cases that require mandatory review by an ethics committee regardless of whether or not there is conflict among the clinicians and family. I believe that an infant bioethics committee should accept cases for review from any hospital employee or staff member, any member of the infant's family or the legal guardian, or any outside agency with relevant interest. I also believe that parents should be fully informed that an ethics committee consultation has been requested, but they should not be permitted to refuse to allow the consultation.

Differing from many commentators, I believe committee review should be mandated for all cases in which it is proposed to withdraw or withhold life-sustaining treatment from any infant who is not imminently dying, regardless of whether there is disagreement among or between clinicians and family members. Review is clearly unnecessary for cases in which withdrawal decisions are being made for infants who are imminently dying or for cases in which withholding decisions are being made for terminally ill infants for whom there are no additional beneficial treatments, unless there is conflict among stakeholders. I believe the decision to require mandatory review of cases when the child is not imminently dying, even when there is no disagreement among family and clinicians, is warranted to protect the interests of infant patients and to provide a level of institutional scrutiny and accountability of neonatal decision-making that did not exist in Bloomington, Indiana, or Stony Brook, New York, when refusal of surgery was allowed for Baby Doe and Baby Jane Doe based on the recommendation of a physician and the agreement of the family. Having participated in the debates and discussions at that time, I believe the public and the state has the right to expect an adequate level of procedural review of decisions that will result in the death of any infant who is not otherwise imminently dying, regardless of whether all caregivers and family members directly involved agree with that course of action. I know this is a minority view, but I am sympathetic with those who believe such decisions should be more transparent and open to additional scrutiny.

Our committee reviewed many cases and, of course, over time developed some methods to streamline the process. Since many neonatal cases in which consideration of whether treatment should be withheld or withdrawn have similar fact patterns and no conflicts, a full committee was not convened for every case. A single member of the committee could consult on these common cases, assure that all the medical facts were clear, and that the family was adequately involved and understood and approved the plan; then the consultant would report back to the full committee at its next meeting. In the first three years of the existence of the committee, we reviewed 10% of the neonatal deaths, which accounted for about 1% of the neonatal intensive care unit admissions. Case review resulted in a recommendation to go to court to reverse parental refusal of surgery in one instance. In every other case, the result of the ethics consultation was the support of the parental decision. Committee members and the staff in the unit all agreed that the committee was extremely helpful to families and staff in clarifying the issues and providing ethical comfort to the decision makers by confirming that the choices made were reasonable and consistent with the best interests of the child. Several studies have shown that infant bioethics committees, like ethics consultations and ethics committees in general, can provide important input into the value laden decisions made in neonatal intensive care units.

ETHICAL ANALYSIS IN NEONATAL INTENSIVE CARE

Virtually all parents love their children, particularly their newborns, and all hope that their children will be healthy. When newborns are critically ill, parents are devastated, and may feel anxious, frightened, angry, guilty, and sad. They are often overwhelmed by the enormity and complexity of the situation, and need help to understand their feelings and to sort out their options. Clinicians should meet regularly with families and keep them apprised of the condition of their child. Physicians and nurses need to be as clear and honest as possible, titrating the information to the needs and desires of each family. Some families will focus on the issues affecting their child now, whereas others may wish to ask a lot of questions about the future. All parents want to know if their baby will survive, when he or she will come home, and if he or she will be "normal."

Parents are thrust into the strange environment of the neonatal intensive care unit. A frightening place where the monitors and intravenous pumps alarm continually, where people speak an incomprehensible language of terms and abbreviations indigenous to this culture, and where babies live or die dependent on the efforts of a rotating group of clinicians of very diverse backgrounds. Doctors and nurses explain the medical facts, as they know them, to parents, and ask them to participate in decision-making for their baby right from the beginning. Parents very quickly realize that they must learn the new language to comprehend their baby's response to his or her illness, and to ask intelligent questions. They also need to understand that much of what they are being told is unclear, not because the persons explaining the information are poor communicators (although that may be the case), but because the information is very complicated. They also learn that short- and long-term predictions about their baby are extremely uncertain.

Dr. and Mrs. Madison, and Mr. and Mrs. Rodriquez, the parents in the two cases described in this chapter, were thrust into a neonatal intensive care unit with virtually no time to prepare for this distressing and chaotic experience. These couples responded differently to the experience of giving birth to a critically ill child, but they both had a clear idea of what they believed would be in the best interest of their child. The Madisons, fearing that their son might survive and be severely impaired, wished to withdraw treatment and allow him to die. The Rodriquez's, hoping for a miracle, refused to give up hope that their son might recover, and asked the doctors to do everything they could to keep him alive. What are the ethical questions raised by these two cases? Are parents the appropriate decision-makers for their neonates, and are there any limits on parental discretion in decision-making? What do parents mean when they say, "do everything"? What are the roles and the obligations of physicians in decision-making for neonates? Does the possibility of a good outcome, however slim, require physicians to advocate for continued treatment? Should physicians refuse to offer treatments that are believed to be only marginally beneficial and only prolong the life of a neonate who will inevitably die? Is there a time when further treatment becomes "futile" for a sick neonate? Is neonatal intensive care for marginally viable infants really "experimental?" Should the costs of continuing treatment be taken into account when making life and death decisions for neonates at the bedside?

Parents are the appropriate decision-makers for health-related choices for their newborns. In our society, we give parents wide latitude to decide what enhances their child's well-being in areas ranging from housing, clothing, nutrition, and religious practices, to healthcare. It can be argued that, more than anyone else, parents have an identity of interests with their children, and an ethical obligation based in beneficence to advocate for their child's best interest. Parental discretion in decision-making is quite broad, but there are some limits. Parents' choices for their children do not hold the same weight as capacitated adults' choices for themselves. Autonomous adults may refuse any medical intervention, even if physicians and family members might feel that those interventions are in the interests of the patient. Parents are not autonomous decision-makers for their children. Parents are surrogate decision-makers, who are not permitted to refuse efficacious treatments when refusal might place their child at imminent risk of irreversible harm. Physicians, and the society at large, have interests in protecting children from harm and assuring that parents are acting responsibly concerning their child's interests.

Healthcare professionals play a major role in assessing what is in the interests of their patients. Particularly in neonatal medicine, where patients cannot make autonomous choices and have never voiced any preferences about treatment, physicians have beneficence-based obligations to advocate for their patients' interests when critical choices must be made. Although physicians should respect the concepts of family-centered care that encourage the involvement of parents in all decisions related to their child, this does not mean that parents should be permitted to make decisions that are clearly against the best interests of their child. Healthcare professionals must make judgements, independent of family wishes, concerning what they believe is the right choice for their patient. Physicians stand as societal representatives to assure that the choices parents make for their children are within the range of acceptable options and based on a reasonable assessment of the interests of the child.

Clinicians and parents may sometimes disagree about what course of action to take for a critically ill child. This is often based on two differing perceptions of what is in the best interest of the child. Dr. and Mrs. Madison believed that their son Joey's death was in his interest, because of his present suffering and grim future prognosis. They also had feelings about how Joey's life might impact on their own lives and on the lives of future children they hoped to conceive. Dr. Kaufman disagreed with the Madisons' view of Joey's best interest. He believed that it was in Joey's interest to continue aggressive treatment. He knew that Joey might die or have a very poor future quality of life, but he also knew that sometimes children like Joey do well. Therefore, he believed he was obligated to advocate for further treatment. These disagreements are often based on uncertain prognosis due to current evidence about outcome, or on differences in valuing the potential for a poor future quality of life. Physicians are not obligated to advocate for aggressive treatment if there is only a slim possibility of a good outcome. Physicians should accept that parents may have a differing view of the best interest of the patient, and that it is acceptable for families to choose to not impose marginally beneficial interventions on their child.

Both parents and professionals bring personal values to the assessment of the child's interests. Professionals need to assist parents to explore their views and values, help them to express their feelings, and to understand that while trying to place the patient's interests as the primary focus of the decision, it is impossible to separate the decision from its impact on the lives and interests of other loved family members. The complexity and serious nature of these decisions requires an in-depth look at the multiplicity of concerns that enter into the final choice.

Physicians also bring personal values and experiences to the recommendations they provide to families. Some physicians wish to arrogate to themselves these hard decisions, believing that they are the best person to make the choice. Some are worried that they will be criticized or sued for allowing a child to die. Others are concerned that the death of a child is a failure. And still others have strongly held religious beliefs that motivate their actions. It is important that clinicians explore their own values and feelings, assess their motivation, and try to place the interests of the child as the primary focus of their recommendations and actions. Most physicians are comfortable with respecting the wishes of parents in cases when it is unclear what is in the interests of the patient. Although clinicians may disagree with a parent's perception of what is the right choice for a critically ill child, they should maintain respect for the parent's views and values. Clinicians must keep in mind that reasonable people may disagree concerning what is the right choice in a complex case, and that respect for an opinion and deference to the right of the parent to make the decision does not imply agreement.

In the United States today, decision-making for critically ill children is a shared activity between parents and healthcare professionals. Although parents generally have the ultimate authority to make these decisions, clinicians must provide the needed medical information, make recommendations about what treatments are medically indicated and will be offered to the child, and assist in the assessment of what is in the interests of the child. Historically, physicians made these decisions, paternalistically imposing their views on families. After several decades of discussion, families won the right to allow their children to die by withholding or withdrawing medical treatments. It was rare that families and physicians disagreed about continuing treatment for a sick child. Disagreement primarily revolved around stopping treatment. With enhancing technology and decreasing mortality in neonatal units, more infants are neurologically devastated yet able to be kept alive on respirators with little hope of reversal of the underlying illness. Clinicians, who have accepted the right of parents to allow their children to die, are now more often faced with parents who demand that their children continue to live.

Increasingly, clinicians are concerned that families like the Rodriquez's in Case 2, are asking them to continue treatment when the prognosis is grim. Physicians and nurses feel a great deal of moral distress as they become the agents of the continued suffering of a patient with no hope for reversal of a devastating illness or reasonable future quality of life. Parents often ask clinicians to "do everything" for their baby. What do they mean? Parents generally do not know all the possible therapies and treatments available to their infants. They invoke this type of language to symbolize their request that the clinicians provide all treatments that might be of help to their child. Clinicians, then, need to make a distinction between everything that is in their armamentarium, and all the treatments that are medically indicated and potentially beneficial for this child. There is never an obligation to do everything, only to do those things that are potentially helpful. Also, doing everything may have a time-limited component. Parents may wish to provide all types of treatments that might be helpful, but only for a certain period of time, after which they would consider withholding or withdrawing them.

Many parents, like the Rodriquez family, invoke their religious beliefs or the hope for a miracle as the reason to request continued treatment. They ask that the doctors and nurses continue to support their child so that God may heal their child and make him well. Many faiths believe that God can cure, or that God works through doctors and nurses to heal the sick. When health professionals are the agent of God's action, the hoped for miracle appears to be one of allowing time to heal the child's illness, despite the poor prognosis, rather than a sudden divine intervention to change the health of the child. Belief in spiritualism and religious forces greater than science and medicine to intervene in illness are values held by many individuals and families. These values deserve our respect, even though they can result in continuing treatment of a child when death or severe disability is likely. Engaging the family in a discussion of their religious and spiritual beliefs and inviting their religious leaders to pray at the bedside or at another location in the neonatal unit can be helpful to convince the family that clinicians accept and respect their belief systems.

If a treatment cannot benefit a patient, it should be considered futile and healthcare professionals have no obligation to provide it. However, physicians often use the term futile or nonbeneficial to describe a treatment that is unlikely to cure or enhance the future quality of a patient's life. The use of the term *futile* should be reserved for those treatments that cannot work in the strict physiologic sense. A respirator for a patient who is not breathing is rarely futile. It may provide only marginal benefit to the long term outcome of the patient, may be prolonging dying, may be increasing suffering, and may not be in the patient's interest, but it is not physiologically futile if it is able to assist in oxygenation and ventilation. Physicians may not wish to provide such treatments based on their perception of the best interest of their patient and may even wish to opt out of the care of such a patient by transferring care to another physician; but they should not invoke the language of futility when they mean that a treatment is only marginally beneficial.

Several hospitals and at least one state, Texas, have attempted to codify a process that may provide guidance to physicians faced with what they believe to be inappropriate requests for continued treatment of terminally ill and incapacitated patients receiving life-sustaining treatments. These approaches are invoked when the treating physician believes that continued provision of life-sustaining treatment is not medically and ethically indicated based on an assessment of what is in the patient's interest, a belief that such treatment will not benefit the patient and will merely prolong an inevitable dying process. An ethics committee must review each of these cases. The surrogate decision-maker or family members must be informed that the review is occurring and, in most cases, may attend the committee meeting. The committee is charged with first attempting to mediate the conflict to come to some reasonable plan about treatment for the patient. If this is not possible, and if the committee concurs with the physician's assessment that life-sustaining treatment is inappropriate and the surrogate decision-maker continues to desire treatment, the physician may seek to transfer the care of the patient to another willing physician or facility. If no such willing physician or facility can be found, according to Texas law, life-sustaining treatment may be stopped after ten days.

The Texas law makes no attempt to define futile treatments. It requires a process that identifies which treatments are not medically indicated, sometimes based on value-laden judgments. Many commentators have argued that this process makes the hospital ethics committee too powerful and may result in discrimination against vulnerable patients and families. The law gives legal safe haven to clinicians and the hospital, and it alleviates the moral distress of clinicians caused by continued treatment of infants like Juan Rodriquez, our second case. But it allows the physician and other individuals outside the family to impose their values, while not respecting the values and religious beliefs of the family members. This approach may be argued to be better than the status quo, if we accept that family members do not have the best interest of their infants at heart when they advocate for prolonging life in the face of what the medical profession believes is significant suffering and inevitable death. But I believe the potential for abuse of this process by powerful physicians whose values differ from those of their patient's family is considerable.

Sometimes when parents and clinicians disagree about withdrawing treatments from a child to allow him to die, it is not about two differing views of the best interest of the child. Sometimes parents will explain that they know their child is critically ill and unlikely to survive, but they just cannot be the ones who will make the decision that results in the death of their child. It is very important for clinicians to hear and appreciate the importance of this language. Physicians must share the burden of the decision with these parents. This can be accomplished by laying out a plan of management for the child and obtaining acquiescence from the parents, rather than by affirmative consent. Rather than the language of "would you like us to . . .," physicians should explain that "we plan to. . . .," and then pause for the parents' response. Clearly, if parents object to the proposed plan, then clinicians may not proceed with it, but if parents accept a plan that might include withholding additional medications or not attempting resuscitation in the event of the heart stopping, then physicians may implement that course of action. This approach is not disingenuous; it is sensitive to the needs and values of some families.

It is also the responsibility of the physician to decide which treatments are medically indicated and offered to the family. Dialysis in response to kidney failure, cardiac medications in response to a failing heart, abdominal surgery in response to a perforated bowel, neurosurgery in response to increasing fluid in the brain, may be possible interventions, but they are not medically indicated when a patient will die in a short time regardless of the treatment or when the treatment will hasten the death rather than prevent it. Treatments that are not medically indicated should not be offered to patients. Physicians do not need permission from families to not offer or to not provide interventions that are not medically indicated. Such treatments merely increase suffering and prolong dying.

THE WINDOW OF OPPORTUNITY

There is a specific group of patients in neonatal intensive care suffering from birth asphyxia for whom decisions about withdrawal of life support are particularly difficult. These infants are often born at term and sustain sudden, unpredicted, fetal distress with lack of oxygen resulting in severe brain injury. At the time of birth, significant brain swelling occurs that affects the ability to breathe and requires ventilatory support. Prognosis for recovery is often uncertain. Over the next three to five days, as brain swelling decreases, the infant may begin to breath on his own, no longer dependent on life support. During that same time, the child may develop clear signs of devastating and irreversible brain damage. Thus, there is a brief window of opportunity during a period of physiologic instability, when withdrawal of treatment will result in the death of the child. If the decision to withdraw treatment is delayed until there is greater prognostic certainty, the opportunity to allow the child to die may no longer exist. Despite the recent promotion of brain cooling immediately after birth as a neuro-protective intervention that may decrease long-term brain damage, almost half of the infants with severe birth asphyxia will die in the neonatal period or survive with severe impairments. Thus, in this situation, unlike most others, there is urgency to confront the difficult decision about continuing life-sustaining treatment.

The term itself, *window of opportunity*, seems a bit ghoulish, suggesting that death is opportune and implying a desire to hasten death. This has resulted in the recommendation, by some, to not inform families about this issue. However, if one agrees that an assessment of the future quality of life of the infant is a relevant and important part of parental decision-making about withdrawal of life-sustaining treatments, and if the opportunity to make the decision to allow the child to die is significantly time limited, then it seems reasonable that parents should be informed about this physiologic period of instability and their options about continuing ventilatory support. Others argue, that if the child has severe brain damage, but is able to breathe on his own, he will likely require artificially provided fluids and nutrition because of an inability to suck and swallow normally. Theoretically, medically provided food and hydration may be withdrawn, allowing the child to die later while breathing on its own. Thus, if discussion of this issue is avoided there is still the possibility to withdraw treatment and allow the child to die in the subsequent weeks. Withdrawal of medically provided food and fluids in infants is very controversial and a difficult choice for most families and clinicians. Although I believe this type of withdrawal of treatment is ethically justifiable, it is far less common and less likely to occur.

Thus, it seems reasonable to discuss these issues with parents soon after the birth of a severely asphyxiated neonate. Although I do not recommend using the term *window of opportunity*, I do believe clinicians should explain to the family that their child is seriously ill from having suffered a severe insult to his brain and other organs that has resulted in the need for ventilatory support. It is important to set out a plan, in consultation with neurologic colleagues, for evaluation and imaging during the first day of life to help clarify the extent of irreversible brain damage, and to offer therapeutic brain cooling and seizure medications if appropriate. On the second day of life, another meeting with the family can address what is known and the best estimates about prognosis based on the child's evolving clinical condition and brain imaging. At that point, withdrawal of life sustaining treatment can be discussed if warranted, and the fact that the child may begin to breathe within the next few days as the swelling decreases should be mentioned. It is difficult, but important, to explain to the family that the resumption of breathing, a result of reversal of brain stem malfunction, may seem like a good sign, but it also may be associated with devastating and irreversible upper brain damage. Although most families need time to digest all this information and to make a thoughtful decision about their child's future, physicians should share their sense of urgency about the need to make a decision and offer to be available for further discussion over the ensuing hours and days. As always, physicians need to reassure families that they will support whatever decision they make, that some loving parents have been in favor of continuing aggressive treatments, whereas other loving families have decided to forego treatments in favor of comfort measures and have allowed their child to die. I have assisted families with decision-making during this window of opportunity. It is not easy, but it is important in order to permit them to have the full range of information needed to make informed choices for their very sick newborn.

IS NEONATAL CARE EXPERIMENTAL?

For years, some commentators have argued that neonatal intensive care is experimental. With all of its risky treatments and uncertain outcomes, it is not surprising that some people think neonatal care should be provided with the oversight of the research regulatory structure. This argument has primarily been invoked to empower parents with the right to refuse to have their children exposed to the risky technological interventions of uncertain outcome used in neonatal intensive care. Participation in clinical research has always been viewed as optional and requires the full and informed consent of the patient or, in the case of children, of the parent or legal guardian. Clinical interventions that are experimental require review and approval by institutional review committees, must provide a clear informed-consent process, and may be refused without question. The goal of research is to ascertain whether a clinical intervention is effective, and whether the benefits outweigh the risks. This basic uncertainty as to outcome makes all research optional, with no obligation to participate.

Although many interventions in the neonatal intensive care unit are high risk, and some have a low likelihood of success, most have been subjected to experimental verification and have known levels of effectiveness and risk. Thus, neonatal care, per se, ought not be considered clinical research. This does not mean that parents ought not have the right to decide whether they wish their child to receive risky clinical interventions. Clinicians are obligated to explain treatment plans to parents and to obtain their permission to proceed with risky interventions that are of low likelihood to succeed.

COST AND NEONATAL CARE

Inevitably, many commentators considering the ethics of continued treatment of critically ill neonates raise the question of the economic costs of these babies to society. They argue that a fair distribution of healthcare resources should invoke the principle of distributive justice and obligate sacrifice of a few for the benefit of many. Are there infants whose care costs so much and their outcomes are so poor that society should not expend the resources to save them? It is estimated that the total annual cost of neonatal care in the United States is over $10 billion per year. Individual sick neonates often cost hundreds of thousands of dollars, and a few cost over a million dollars in the first year of life. Are these expenditures justified when there are millions of individuals whose basic healthcare needs are not being met? Should neonates with a prognosis for a poor future quality of life be sacrificed for the benefit of these other societal members?

There are two major problems with these arguments. First, if we accept the premise of the argument, how would we choose which neonates meet the criteria of having a poor future quality of life? And how would these assessments be certain to not discriminate against vulnerable infants and families from minority populations? Second, why are we only talking about neonates? Why are we willing to discuss sacrificing a small number of neonates who generate significant expenditures, rather than looking at the extraordinarily large expenditures being spent on elderly patients who are marginally conscious on respirators in nursing homes, or the costs of treatments that may prolong the lives of cancer patients for a few months, or other expensive treatments for adult populations? When Americans are ready to discuss seriously the appropriateness of providing interventions for all incapacitated and chronically ill patients who will only marginally benefit from these expenditures, then those who advocate for infants should be open to such considerations. Until then, the best-interest approach for neonates, implemented through parental choice with clinician involvement, seems to be the fairest way to assure that the interests of individual infants are appropriately considered.

As the financing of healthcare delivery evolves and accountable care organizations take hold in America, economic incentives will change. Clinicians and hospitals will no longer be paid for treating patients who are ill but, rather, will be responsible for preventing illness and keeping populations healthy. Hospitals will become insurers, making it in their economic interests to prevent prematurity, rather than to offer expensive high-tech treatments of marginal benefit to the long-term outcome of sick neonates. The ethical concerns that this series of events creates are obvious. Will this new approach to healthcare financing create disincentives to provide comprehensive treatments for the sickest patients? And how will that affect the involvement of parents in decision-making? Only time will tell.

FINAL THOUGHTS

Children are generally cherished by their families and valued by the society as future contributing members. Society places the responsibility for the well-being of vulnerable children in the hands of their parents. Healthcare professionals are asked to shepherd and nurture this relationship. Parents and physicians have beneficence-based obligations to children to maximize each child's potential and to minimize harms. Parents are the a priori decision-makers for their children, with a broad range of authority and responsibility. They are obligated to make healthcare decisions for their children that place the child's interests as primary. Our society has an important responsibility to ensure that children are not devalued, neglected, or allowed to die because their parents or their physicians are not concerned with their best interest. Additionally, children should not fear that they will be used solely to fulfill the hopes and desires of others, and inappropriately forced to live burdensome lives of poor quality or inordinate suffering.

Jeff Lyon, in his classic book, *Playing God in the Nursery*, graphically portrays the dilemma that parents and physicians often encounter in neonatal intensive care units: "if it is hard to justify creating blind paraplegics to obtain a number of healthy survivors, it is equally hard to explain to the ghosts of the potentially healthy that they had to die in order to avoid creating blind paraplegics." This tragic trade-off is at the heart of many of the difficult choices made everyday in neonatal care. These decisions are not about abstract cases, but about real sons and daughters, with real names, and serious illnesses. These choices will never be easy, but they are best made by parents, counseled by competent, compassionate physicians who all place the future interests of the child as primary.

ADDITIONAL READINGS

American Academy of Pediatrics Committee on Bioethics, Guidelines on Foregoing Life-Sustaining Medical Treatment. *Pediatr*, 1994; 93 532–536.

Campbell DE, Fleischman AR. The limits of viability: dilemmas, decisions and decision makers. *Am J Perinatol*, 2001; 18:117–127.

Duff RS, Campbell AGM, (1973). Moral and ethical dilemmas in the special care nursery. *N Engl J Med*, 289: 890–894.

Fleischman AR. Bioethical review committees in perinatology. *Clin Perinatol*, 1987; 14: 379–393.

Lyon J. *Playing God in the Nursery*. New York, NY: W.W.Norton, 1985.

President's Commission for the Study of Ethical Problems in Medicine and Biomedical and Behavioral Research. *Deciding to Forego Life-extending Treatment*. Washington DC; 1983

CHAPTER 5

Ethical Issues in Genetic Testing and Screening in Children

> ### Case 1
>
> Linda is a 14-year-old girl whose aunt and grandmother died of breast cancer at relatively young ages. Her mother decided to be tested for the genes that would predict her risk for breast cancer, and has recently learned that she is positive. Linda would like to know whether she, too, has an increased risk for breast cancer. Dr. Rose, Linda's pediatrician, who has been caring for her since her birth, is reluctant to perform the test. She tells Linda and her mother that the American Academy of Pediatrics recommends that predictive testing of children for adult-onset conditions generally should be deferred, unless an intervention initiated in childhood may reduce morbidity or mortality. Linda is a thoughtful, intelligent, and responsible young person. She tells Dr. Rose that she wants the test in order to decrease her own anxiety and so she can get on with her life. Her mother is unsure what is best for Linda, but agrees that Linda should have the test if she wants it.

> ### Case 2
>
> Judy and Kiyung Wong were thrilled when their first-born son Jake seemed perfectly normal and healthy at birth. At Jake's two-week check up, their pediatrician told them that the newborn screening panel, drawn shortly after birth was reported from the state laboratory as

revealing no problems. Everyone was surprised at six months of age when Jake seemed to be developing slower than other children his age. The pediatrician reassured the family that every child develops at a different rate and that there was nothing to be concerned about. But when Jake began to have some neurologic symptoms at 9 months of age and was not reaching normal developmental milestones, the pediatrician referred the family to a pediatric neurologist for evaluation. The neurologist diagnosed developmental delay and recommended a series of tests including an EEG and a brain MRI. These tests did not reveal any specific findings or suggest any specific diagnosis. At 15 months of age, the neurologist noted that there was deterioration in Jake's condition, and referred the family to a metabolic expert at the regional medical center for further evaluation. Extensive metabolic testing revealed a rare disease for which there is no known treatment.

Judy and Kiyung were deeply concerned and somewhat confused because they remembered the reassurance that their pediatrician had given them about Jake's newborn screening test. The metabolic expert honestly explained to Judy and Kiyung that Jake's illness could have been detected through newborn screening. In most states, the disease is detected through testing and the information is shared with families, but in their state, even though the test is done as part of newborn screening, the results are not revealed to families because there is no effective treatment available. Kiyung became angry while Judy began to cry. The Wongs sorrow and anger were compounded by the realization that Judy was seven months pregnant and their second baby might have the same problem as Jake.

Case 3

George is the 2-year-old son of Phyllis and Jay Brandon. He has been exhibiting developmental delay with some concern about autism because of poor ability to interact with his environment and with his parents. The Brandons have been taking George for care at a major academic medical center. The pediatricians at the center offer the family whole exome testing for George in the hope that they will find a genetic mutation that is responsible for his problems. The doctors explain that the testing may not reveal a specific genetic diagnosis nor a treatment that will help George, but it may give the family some insight into his problem. Over time, with testing of other children who have a similar genetic mutation, possible treatments and better prediction of prognosis may evolve. They also explained to the Brandons that there is the possibility that genomic testing may reveal other genetic mutations not related to autism and developmental delay. Phyllis and Jay agree that whole exome testing is the right thing to do for George.

Test results reveal no known genetic abnormalities related to autism or developmental delay, but they do find genetic mutations that are associated with increased risk for breast cancer and early-onset Alzheimer's disease.

BACKGROUND

Many diseases run in families and seem to have an inherited component. The field of genetics is the study of our heredity and the potential for each of us to pass on certain traits and characteristics biologically to our offspring through reproduction. For over 150 years we have known that traits could be inherited, and in the early 20th century we learned of the existence of chromosomes present in the nucleus of cells that were the vectors of our heredity. But only in the last 60 years have we learned of the characteristics of the genetic material, DNA, the biologic substrate found in chromosomes that makes this possible.

The specific sequence of chemical base pairs that make up double-stranded human DNA was defined through a major international research collaboration, the Human Genome Project, completed in 2003. This initiated the modern era of "genetic medicine." From the perspective of our genomes, all humans are more alike than different, with over 99% of our DNA being identical. Less than one percent of the genome differentiates each human as unique.

The totality of the DNA provides an "instruction manual" that informs each cell in the body how to function. Although there are about 3 billion individual chemical bases that make up the genome, there are only about 20,000 actual genes. Each gene is programmed to create RNA, a mirror image of the DNA, in order to produce a specific protein needed for cellular function. If a gene is damaged because it has a missing base or a different base substituted for the correct one, it may be unable to create the needed protein, or it may create an abnormal protein, or too much protein. These changes in genes are called mutations and generally have insignificant impact on health and well-being. But some genetic mutations are responsible for serious, although generally rare, diseases. Since DNA is double stranded, a single mutation on one of the strands most often does not result in any functional problem, but it allows that normal person carrying a mutation to pass it on to future offspring. When each member of a procreating couple is a carrier of a genetic mutation in the same gene, they may both pass the abnormal gene to their offspring, resulting in an affected child. Mutations in the same gene can vary greatly. This results in wide variation in the severity and presenting symptoms, or "phenotype" of a disease. Thus, a single genetic disorder may manifest very differently in different people.

The era of genetic medicine has resulted in the identification of hundreds of single gene disorders that cause significant disease, and the development of modern technologies to sequence the genome faster and at lower cost. Studies of the genetic makeup of individuals with complex conditions such as diabetes, heart disease, and autism reveal that these conditions are caused by the interaction of multiple genes along with the influence of a myriad of environmental, social, and behavioral factors. Additional scientific discoveries expanded understanding of the role and regulation of genes. It is now believed that genes may produce more than one protein and can be controlled and regulated by interactions with genomic and nongenomic factors. Various environmental chemicals, regulatory proteins, and specific RNA molecules interact to turn genes on and off and regulate gene function. These observations have helped in the understanding of the pathogenesis and treatment of diseases as diverse as cancer, autism, and AIDS, ushering in a new era of genomic medicine.

Whole genome testing is now available as a clinical tool for patients with undefined disorders, and has also been offered directly to the public as a way of exploring risk of future disease. Whole genome sequencing is marketed to healthy individuals who wish to understand more about their personal risk of developing single gene disorders that present later in life, as well as their risk of complex conditions not defined by a single gene. Whole genome sequencing has also been recommended for children with signs or symptoms that are suggestive of a specific genetic disorder but for whom the known disease gene does not contain any mutation, and for children with unique phenotypes that have not previously been associated with a single gene defect. Although it is possible to sequence the entire genome, most clinical laboratories choose to examine a much smaller portion of the genome, those parts of the DNA that are known to code for proteins, the exome.

Another research tool in the genomic era has been the use of genome-wide association studies to identify genes associated with risk of acquiring a complex condition. Initial studies used "candidate genes" gleaned from the genomes of patients with a specific condition to compare to a sample of patients with that disorder or to a larger group of the public to see if one could associate the development of the condition to carrying one or more of the candidate genes. With the advent of more sophisticated genomic-sequencing technologies and new analytic capacities, novel genetic risk factors can be discovered by testing hundreds of thousands of small portions of the genome from large populations. Although genetic associations have been found for virtually every complex condition that tends to run in families, these genetic components explain a very small proportion of the observed contribution of heredity to the risk of disease, often less than 5%. This suggests that environmental factors play a much larger role in disease causation and variation than was previously expected. Thus, the use of genetic markers to predict risk of such complex conditions has limited, if any, clinical utility.

The genomic era has also seen the advent of personalized medicine with the focus on pharmacogenomics. Recent studies reveal that individual patient response to medications is modulated by genetic factors. Efficacy, toxicity, and drug metabolism may vary widely based on the genetic makeup of the patient. Identifying these genetic factors through carefully crafted clinical trials of new and standard medications will potentially allow physicians to customize medical treatments for individual patients, increasing effectiveness and decreasing idiosyncratic reactions to a prescribed drug.

GENETIC TESTING AND SCREENING

Genetic testing is used clinically in individual children with certain physical characteristics or symptoms that point to a genetic disorder in order to confirm a suspected diagnosis and assist with determining prognosis and treatment. Genetic testing in clinical practice can examine the number and structure of chromosomes in cell nuclei or the specific DNA makeup of individual genes. Chromosomal disorders of extra copies of an entire chromosome, such as exists in Down syndrome, or alterations of a chromosome by a partial deletion or addition of genetic material may be detected in children with developmental delay, unusual appearance, or other abnormalities. An abnormality in a single gene accounting for disease is rare, but single-gene disorders result in a large number of pediatric hospitalizations. In the first decades of the 21st century the ability to examine single-gene disorders has exploded as technology has allowed for more rapid and less expensive analysis of individual gene loci. Single-gene disorders vary from the somewhat more common and well-known diseases, such as cystic fibrosis and sickle cell anemia, to extraordinarily rare disorders of protein metabolism affecting neurodevelopment in only a handful of children. Even single-gene disorders can show wide variations in phenotype and clinical course, owing to various mutations in the abnormal gene or the effect of other genes and environmental factors on gene expression. The clinical utility of genetic testing in individual children with specific signs and symptoms has been proven and is being integrated increasingly into pediatric practice. Defining the specific diagnosis can be extremely helpful to delineate treatment options and characterize prognosis.

Genetic screening differs from testing. Genetic testing is performed on an individual patient when a single-gene disease is suspected. Testing generally reveals a specific and definitive diagnosis, linking a genetic abnormality with signs and symptoms in an individual patient. Genetic screening is performed on individuals or populations who are not symptomatic to find those individuals who or are at risk to develop a genetic disease or to find those who are carriers of genetic material that may be passed on to their offspring through reproduction. Some screening tests for single-gene disorders are performed by measurement of gene products rather than by actual gene testing. Thus, confirmatory gene testing is often required when individuals are suspected of having a genetic disorder from the results of a screening test.

In addition to screening for single-gene disorders, genetic screening can also be done for complex conditions such as heart disease or diabetes. Such screening involves examining multiple genetic markers and provides a probabilistic estimate of the risk for developing a specific disease in the future.

With this brief background on genetics and genomics, we can begin to discuss some ethical questions about genetic information that are relevant to children and their families. Does genetic information determine one's destiny? Is genetic information special and somehow different from other health-related information? If so, should genetic information be treated specially? Can unidentified genetic information be kept anonymous?

Some people believe that genetic information determines a person's physical, behavioral, and social traits as well as their future health and longevity. The term *genetic determinism* was coined to reflect this belief that most human characteristics are preordained by the genetic information programmed into our cells at conception. The belief that our genes fully predict our destiny is naïve and potentially dangerous. Although some genetic information like an additional chromosome or a specific gene mutation can have significant impact on outcome, most genetic information is probabilistic and associated with wide variations in gene expression that is dramatically affected by environmental factors. Thus, social and behavioral factors as well as the chemical and biologic environment affect our genes and determine our ultimate outcome.

Many people believe that genetic information is special, creating ethical concerns unlike those associated with most other medical tests that are important for diagnosis and prognosis of disease. Genetic information for each person is unique and provides a personal identifier. As such, it can never be truly anonymized. However, to actually identify an individual from their genome would require a database of genomes to search. Although the vast majority of individuals have not had their genomes measured and are not in such a database, things are changing. The genome of everyone who enters the military is tested and stored in a federal database. Similarly, the genomes of convicted criminals are measured and stored, and there are an increasing number of research studies and regional biobanks that are accumulating genetic information on healthy individuals and patients. Millions of individuals have had their genomes mapped and much of this information is potentially available at least to law enforcement agencies.

Genetic information is also special because it is relevant not only to the person whose genes are tested, but also to their family members. It is possible that parents, siblings, children, and other close relatives of tested individuals may have a similar genetic composition, sharing a similar risk of disease or transmission of genetic information to offspring. Should a person who learns that they have the risk of a serious genetic disorder share this information with their relatives? Should clinicians urge patients to discuss positive genetic test findings with their close relatives? When knowledge about risk of a future disease can be helpful, like in the case of genetic markers of increased risk of breast cancer, it seems reasonable for individuals to share that knowledge with their close relatives. Similarly, it seems reasonable that clinicians should explain to their patients the relevance of the genetic information to others in the family, encouraging the patient to share this information when appropriate. However, clinicians should respect the privacy and confidentiality of their patients and not reveal results to others without explicit permission.

Like other medical test results, genetic information may engender fear, guilt, anxiety, and social stigma. But because of the future predictive value of genetic information, it is argued that genetic testing is more likely than other medical tests to result in possible insurance and employment discrimination. And, since genetic test results from one individual are likely to have direct implications for others who are genetically related, these other individuals may also be affected by discrimination if those results are known.

Because of the importance and potential impact of genetic information on multiple individuals, the term *"genetic exceptionalism"* was created about 20 years ago.

GENETIC EXCEPTIONALISM

Genetic exceptionalism refers to the belief that genetic information should be treated differently from other medical information. The term was borrowed from similar concerns about how sensitive information related to AIDS should be treated. Because of the highly charged and stigmatizing nature of information related to HIV status, test results, and AIDS diagnosis, "AIDS exceptionalism" argued that all such information should be distinct from other medical information, stored in an extremely confidential manner, and shared with no one without explicit consent. Treating AIDS as exceptional was justified by the fear that individuals and their families would be harmed through violence, isolation, and discrimination if their disease status were revealed. Although AIDS exceptionalism resulted in increased protection of personal privacy, it also had some negative consequences, making HIV testing and partner notification more difficult through complex informed-consent processes and pre- and post-counseling requirements.

Genetic exceptionalism has been justified by the concern that revealing that an individual is at risk for the development of a serious disease could result in significant discrimination in employment and insurance for the person tested and their relatives. If genetic information is to be treated differently from other medical information, what constitutes genetic information? Is genetic information merely the results of chromosome analyses and DNA and RNA assays? Does family history of an inherited disorder or an elevated serum cholesterol level count as genetic information? Concern for genetic exceptionalism and possible discrimination has resulted in the development of state and federal laws that prohibit discrimination in health-insurance coverage and employment based on genetic information. These laws have had to define what constitutes genetic information.

Perhaps the most influential U.S. law is the federal *Genetic Information Nondiscrimination Act (GINA)*, signed into law in 2008. GINA prohibits discrimination in health-insurance coverage and employment based on genetic information. It sets the minimum standards for protection for all Americans, while allowing individual states to develop even more protective laws. A genetic test is defined by the law to include analyses of human DNA, RNA, chromosomes, proteins, or metabolites that detect genotypes, mutations, or chromosomal changes. Routine blood tests such as blood counts, cholesterol levels, or liver function tests are not included in the definition. Genetic information is defined as the results of an individual's genetic test as well as the results of genetic tests from family members up to and including fourth-degree relatives. Genetic tests on family members who are pregnant women and their fetuses and embryos are also included. Family history of a genetic disease and request for genetic counseling services are also included in the definition of genetic information that is protected. GINA also applies to genetic information obtained through participation in a research study.

The protections against discrimination afforded by GINA are not unlimited. Nondiscrimination in health-insurance coverage does not extend to disability, long-term care, or life insurance. The protection against discrimination in health-insurance coverage does not prohibit a health insurer from increasing insurance premiums based on manifestations of a disease or disorder even if genetic in nature. Since employers are increasingly becoming health insurers, it will be important for GINA to be strengthened and clarified in the future to afford greater protections against discrimination in employment and health insurance based on genetic information.

GENETIC SCREENING—UNIQUE ISSUES IN CHILDREN

Genetic testing and screening in adults includes many ethical concerns that can be addressed through the process of informed consent. Adults seeking knowledge about genetic disease, predictive information about their future risk for illness, or the potential to pass genetic traits or diseases to their offspring generally have the capacity to give informed consent for the testing. Adults are presumed to have the ability to evaluate the risks and benefits of genetic testing after receiving an adequate amount of information provided in a clear and understandable manner and followed by an open discussion to answer any concerns or questions. On the other hand, children, particularly infants and young children, are not able to evaluate the risks and benefits of testing and provide informed consent. This is not a problem when there is a clear and direct benefit to the child of testing. Parents may give consent for clinically relevant tests for their children as they would for all other medical tests and treatments. But, should parents be allowed to consent for tests that are only predictive of future risk of adult-onset diseases for which there are no interventions or treatments that can prevent or ameliorate the disease? Should newborn screening for genetic disorders require parental consent? Should parents be allowed to consent for tests that may predict risk of their child becoming violent, alcoholic, or homosexual—behaviors that may manifest in childhood?

Predictive genetic testing of children based on family history of disorders that display age-dependent penetrance (appearing in adulthood) has been strongly discouraged unless there are effective interventions that can be initiated in childhood to prevent or ameliorate future morbidity and mortality. This approach has been justified based on respect of the child's future autonomy and protection of the child's choice about whether he or she wants to know the information. Since the child will not receive treatments or interventions to prevent or ameliorate the disease, pediatric and genetic professionals have refused to offer such testing or comply with parental requests for testing. They argue that children should be allowed to make this choice for themselves when they become adults. Some commentators have questioned this absolutist approach, arguing that contextual factors should be taken into account and that a more individualized approach might be warranted. Although agreeing that young children cannot make informed choices about such complex issues, they argue that many adolescents are capable of assessing their own interests and, particularly in the context of a familial disease and the possibility of reproductive choices being thrust upon them, should be allowed to consent to predictive genetic testing for themselves.

The American Academy of Pediatrics, mirroring many other thoughtful organizations with interest in genetics, recommends that "predictive genetic testing (of children and adolescents) for adult onset conditions generally should be deferred unless an intervention initiated in childhood may reduce morbidity or mortality. An exception might be made for families for whom diagnostic uncertainty poses a significant psychosocial burden, particularly when an adolescent and his or her parents concur in their interest in predictive testing." They recommend that, in general, pediatricians should decline requests from parents to obtain predispositional genetic testing until the child has the capacity to make the choice.

Pediatric and genetic organizations justify the recommendation not to offer families genetic testing for late-onset diseases for their children and to decline to provide testing if requested, based on the concern that knowing the results of the test does not always result in a good outcome, particularly when there are no interventions that can be initiated in childhood to prevent or ameliorate the disease, and when such results merely provide probabilistic data. Many adults choose not to be tested for risk of adult-onset disease that runs in their family because of the fear that knowing may cause undue anxiety and stress, and significant depression. Other adults choose to be tested because they believe knowing they are at risk will help them cope, and learning they are not at risk will relieve their anxiety about the future.

Linda, the 14-year-old girl in Case 1 whose grandmother and aunt have died of breast cancer and whose mother has just tested positive for a gene that places her at a significantly increased risk of cancer, argues that she is well aware of the benefits and risks of testing, since she observed her mother's process of decision-making and her mother's response to the positive results. She has convinced her parents that, for her, knowing is preferable to waiting. The pediatrician, Dr. Rose, is reluctant to allow testing, based on her concern that Linda will decompensate and become terribly depressed if the result is positive. Dr. Rose fears that Linda's rational argument in favor of testing is based on the subconscious belief that the test will be negative, and on an inadequate understanding of the powerful impact a positive test may have on her psychological well being.

This is a truly difficult ethical dilemma. The ethical questions to be considered include the following: Does this fourteen-year-old girl have the capacity to make this decision? Should decisions by adolescents be given the same respect as those made by adults? If the child and the family agree that testing is in the child and family's best interest, should the pediatrician refuse to participate in that choice? Should the state make laws or regulations that would preclude the family from obtaining Linda's blood test to determine whether she is at increased risk for an adult-onset genetic disease?

As we will explore further in the chapter on adolescents, many 14-year-olds have the capacity to assess the benefits and burdens of difficult health-related choices. Their decisions appear to be as well thought out as those of adults. That isn't to say that adults always make the best choices for themselves, but 14-year-olds appear to be as good at making hard choices related to their health care as adults. Teens, however, do tend to be more optimistic about their futures, and tend to trivialize the negative consequences of their actions more than adults. Dr. Rose's concern that Linda is not being realistic about the effects of a positive result is certainly important. Dr. Rose will need to frankly explore these concerns with Linda in a private setting where she can assess whether Linda is being unduly influenced by her parents' views and whether Linda has a good understanding of the consequences of her choice. Dr. Rose should also share her concerns with Linda's parents to gauge their insight into the potential negative consequences of a positive test result. Dr. Rose may also wish to explore how Linda's mother is responding to her own positive test result, and how she will counsel Linda if she is also found to test positive.

Although many organizations have recommended that children not be tested for adult-onset diseases until they can make autonomous choices for themselves, there are no state laws that preclude such testing. I beleive that each of these cases needs to be considered in the full context of the family history, parental views, and the child's ability to make a truly informed choice. Dr. Rose may ethically choose to refuse to be involved in prescribing the test because of her personal assessment of what is in the best interest of Linda, but the family will likely be able to obtain the test either from another doctor or through the many direct-to-consumer genetic testing services that exist today. If Dr. Rose believes that Linda and her family have assessed the risks and benefits of the testing and have concluded that testing is best for Linda, I believe that Dr. Rose should agree to perform the test. This would allow Dr. Rose to maintain a close relationship with Linda and her family and to supply post-test counseling and needed support, regardless of the result.

Newborn Screening

Increasingly, genetic testing is being used to presymptomatically diagnose a disease or to predict the risk that a disorder will develop. This type of testing can be performed on entire populations, as in the case of screening of all newborns shortly after birth.

Newborn screening is a population-based public health program that utilizes genetic testing or gene-product analysis to provide early identification of rare genetic, metabolic, and hormonal disorders that, without treatment, can have devastating health consequences and, in some cases, lead to death. What began in the mid-1960s as an activity to identify a single rare, but serious, metabolic disease that occurred in about 1 in 25,000 newborns, phenylketonuria, has dramatically expanded. This increase in recent years is primarily due to the advent of new technology, tandem mass spectrometry, to reliably identify abnormal levels of gene products associated with rare genetic disorders. A 2005 report by the American College of Medical Genetics, commissioned by the U.S. Health Resources and Services Administration recommended mandatory newborn screening for a core panel of 29 disorders in an attempt to move the nation toward a uniform newborn screening panel for serious disorders for which effective preventive interventions and treatments exist.

Each state has the legal authority to run its own newborn screening program. All four million babies born in the United States each year have a few drops of blood obtained by heel prick during the first few days of life in the hospital. These drops are placed in circles (spots) on a special filter paper and forwarded to a laboratory for testing. At present, the U.S. newborn screening program identifies over 5,000 children per year with treatable metabolic, hematologic, or hormonal disorders. Laboratory testing requires a very small amount of the sample that is obtained in the first few day of life, so residual blood spots remain after the screening process.

Although the recommended panel of screened disorders has been somewhat controversial, there is more agreement on the principles that should be fulfilled before a disorder becomes part of newborn screening:

- The disorder should be serious and significantly impair health beginning in infancy.
- The test must be performed on blood collected on filter paper shortly after birth, so that it can identify the disorder before the child becomes symptomatic.
- The test must be valid, reliable, sensitive and specific, and able to be performed at a reasonable cost.
- Testing should be mandatory so that every baby will be screened regardless of parental consent.
- There should be evidence that early detection and treatment will provide medical benefit to the affected infant.

The last two principles, the mandatory nature of testing and the requirement that there be a documented medical benefit of early detection and treatment, have met with some controversy. Critics have argued that newborn screening should not be mandatory and should require parental consent, like virtually all other medical testing and treatment decisions for children. Although testing is routinely performed in all states, most states permit parents to opt out or refuse testing of their newborn based on strongly held religious or other beliefs. The justification for not requiring any form of affirmative consent includes the seriousness and rarity of the disorders, the ability to identify a disorder before the child is symptomatic, and the availability of beneficial treatment that must be provided early in infancy to prevent devastating disease.

Those that oppose the mandatory nature of the program argue that although courts have held that parents are not allowed to refuse known efficacious treatments for life- threatening conditions without which the child will suffer imminent and irreversible harm or possibly death, this standard does not apply to screening tests. So critics conclude that parents should be thoroughly informed about newborn screening and given the opportunity to consent or refuse participation. Studies reveal that parents clearly prefer being fully informed about newborn screening and, overwhelmingly, would consent to the testing if asked. Whether to mandate newborn screening without parental consent and whether any parent ought to be allowed to opt out of testing for religious or other reasons remain important ethical questions.

The principle of "parens patriae" or "the state as parent" argues that there is a compelling state interest in protecting the health of children and a state obligation to ensure reasonable behavior on the part of parents to provide adequate medical care for their children. Invoking this doctrine, and through court involvement, states can prevent parents from refusing medical treatments that are known to be effective in preventing imminent harm, irreversible damage, or death to their child. Every state in the United States interprets its obligation to protect children to include testing of all newborns, without parental consent, for at least a basic core panel of disorders. Although consent is not required, in all but one or two states, parents are permitted to refuse testing.

To justify universal screening, all screened disorders are supposed to have evidence of medical benefit from early detection and treatment. All core disorders on the panel of tests in newborn screening are thought to have medical interventions that can directly benefit the affected child. However, some of the positive results in the screening process are for disorders that do not have a medical intervention that has been documented to provide benefit. These disorders are "secondary" conditions that are identified as a result of the use of tandem mass spectrometry as the laboratory approach to newborn screening. Tandem mass spectrometry testing is used to measure 20 of the core conditions. This approach can occasionally reveal results for other known rare and serious disorders for which effective treatment is not available. These additional conditions, revealed as incidental findings of the testing procedure or as a consequence of clarifying the differential diagnosis of a core panel condition, have no effective treatment and do not meet the criteria for mandatory testing.

Because these additional conditions that have no effective treatments are revealed through newborn screening, some believe that parents should be required to consent for newborn screening, or, at a minimum, be informed that these secondary conditions may be found at the time of testing and asked if they wish to be informed about these results if positive. Other commentators conclude that states have an ethical obligation not to reveal these results to families. They argue that the potential harm done by revealing an incidental finding to a family without the availability of treatment is so great as to mandate that states either suppress the information, not revealing it to families, or develop an informed consent that is signed at the time of obtaining the blood sample, allowing families to opt out of learning about positive test results.

This is the problem faced by Judy and Kiyung Wong and their first child Jake in Case 2. During his first year of life, the Wongs observed a slow but continual neurologic deterioration in their son. They sought help first from their pediatrician, then they were referred to a neurologist, and finally they saw a metabolic expert for further evaluation. When Jake was 15 months old and Judy 7-months pregnant with their second child, they learned that Jake was suffering from an inherited rare metabolic disorder for which there is no treatment. The expert who diagnosed Jake's disease mentioned to the family that the newborn screening program in their state chooses not to inform families of disorders for which there is no effective treatment even when the screening test reveals such secondary or incidental findings. The Wongs were devastated by the fact that Jake had a serious and likely fatal disease, but they were also confused and angry that the state had withheld information known about their child. The Wongs felt that their prolonged search for answers as Jake became increasingly ill was unnecessary and expensive. Worse, had they known about Jake's diagnosis, preimplantation genetic testing before pregnancy or amniocentesis during pregnancy would have allowed them to determine if their second child will suffer from the same disease; this could have offered them choices about initiating or continuing the pregnancy.

The issue of whether physicians and researchers should reveal incidental findings to patients or research participants is not new. In the case of newborn screening, most families report wanting to know such information in order to best prepare for the onset of symptoms and to obviate the need for what has been called the diagnostic odyssey, the journey to seek an explanation that families embark on when their child begins to have nonspecific symptoms. Because the diseases are rare and the symptoms not specific, this process can often be protracted and expensive as symptoms worsen. In addition, another pregnancy may ensue without proper preconception testing of the parents that might reveal important information about their reproductive choices and could ensure that their next child is not affected by the same disorder. Virtually all parents of affected children, whether treatment is available or not, indicate that they would have wished to know about the diagnosis prior to initiation of symptoms in infancy. For these reasons, I believe that revealing incidental test results of secondary conditions to families, accompanied by the provision of counseling and support services, seems reasonable. States should not withhold significant health-related information from families about their children. Revealing positive test results also allows families to decide if they wish to consent to enrolling their child in clinical research studies that might be available to explore new potential treatments for that child's disease.

Rather than routinely revealing these incidental findings, some argue that there should be an informed-consent process at the time of obtaining the sample, and it should be designed solely to highlight the potential to learn about incidental test results for secondary conditions. This would be confusing to families at best and could result in more families opting out of the entire newborn-screening process. This could be potentially harmful to many children and their families.

The debate about revealing positive findings of secondary conditions raises a question about whether newborn screening panels ought to include many more devastating disorders for which there are no effective treatments. As new genomic testing technologies become available, it will be possible to test for hundreds of disorders. Even now, some states screen for additional conditions not routinely recommended. This has generally been the result of local efforts by affected families and others who convince state legislatures to mandate testing for a rare and serious disorder even though no effective treatment is available. Well-intentioned legislators have created laws to mandate testing for these additional conditions based on the seriousness of the disorders, but these laws ignore the principles that justify universal mandatory newborn screening. In order to maintain fidelity to the basic principles of newborn screening and to preclude serious criticism from many who do not agree with mandatory testing, if states do add additional tests to their newborn-screening program it is preferable to inform parents at the time of testing that such tests are available on a voluntary basis and obtain their preference before performing such tests.

Even though it is generally believed that informed consent is not required for newborn-screening programs, it is agreed that there is a need for education of families and professionals about newborn screening. It is important to inform all prospective and new parents about newborn screening, its purpose, and the need for immediate confirmatory testing and follow-up if results are positive.

Newborn Screening—Use of Residual Blood Spots

Newborn-screening filter-paper specimens sent to the laboratory contain a very small amount of blood, but more than is required for routine testing. The extra blood is available if there is any question about the results that require repeating as well as for confirmatory testing and quality-control measures. In almost all cases, residual blood spots remain after the screening is completed.

For many years, states have stored residual blood spots for months and even years. During the last 5–10 years, controversy over the fate of the residual blood spots has arisen. In several states, lawsuits were launched by parent groups against public-health agencies over privacy concerns stemming from the use of the samples after screening was completed. The state health departments in Minnesota and Texas were sued in recent years by families who objected to any storage or use of residual specimens without explicit informed consent from parents.

There is wide variation among state regulations and practices concerning the length of storage and postscreening uses of the residual blood spots. Residual blood spots have various uses:

- Test result verification, quality assurance of laboratory testing, and test validation if there is a question in the future about a positive or negative result.
- Development of new, better, or less expensive laboratory methods to screen for currently tested disorders.
- Development of new tests to screen for disorders not currently tested.
- Parental requests for additional testing—particularly in cases of an unexplained death of an infant or young child.
- Forensic or other legal uses including criminal investigations and identification of a missing or kidnapped child.
- Anonymous population-based epidemiologic research after the blood spots are completely separated from all personal identifiers—often used to identify the population prevalence of new infectious agents and toxins passed from mother to baby.
- De-identified population-based epidemiologic research with the potential for re-identification of the subject if the research reveals information of clinical relevance that could impact the health of an individual child or family.
- Clinical research using personal health information—particularly in the case of a child found to have a rare disorder not routinely tested in the core panel of newborn screening who might be referred to clinical trials or longitudinal studies of that disorder.

From an ethical perspective, a clear distinction needs to be made between the uses of residual blood spots that are directly related to the testing program and aim to improve newborn screening as a public-health program and other potential uses of residual blood spots. Newborn-screening programs have generally considered the use of residual blood spots for quality assurance, test validation, and the development of new laboratory methods as integral to the program, thus not requiring any additional consideration of consent from families.

Completely anonymized samples used for the development and validation of new tests for disorders proposed as candidates for newborn screening and similar population-based studies with residual blood spots completely and permanently separated from all personal identifiers do not create any risk of privacy infringement. These types of studies are not considered human subjects research according to the Department of Health and Human Services Office for Human Research Protections and, therefore, should not require informed consent.

A parental request for additional testing of blood spots certainly requires consent and is generally part of clinical or postmortem medical practice. Forensic uses of residual blood spots in criminal investigations have been allowed by some states and have created a great deal of public concern about privacy issues. At a minimum, such uses should require court involvement. I believe that all other uses of residual blood spots with the potential for identification of individual subjects is considered "human subjects research" and should be subject to federal regulations for research with human subjects. All such research is subject to review and approval by state, university, or hospital institutional review boards that are responsible for the protection of human subjects of research. These boards must determine the appropriate mechanism for informing subjects and families about the research and obtaining their consent when required.

States have an obligation to inform families of their intentions concerning the storage and use of residual blood specimens and to obtain permission from families if a use other than test verification, development, or quality assurance is anticipated. A process of opting-in or opting-out of the storage of samples can be ethically justified in most cases, but if samples will be provided to researchers for studies that require personal identifiers, whether linked or unlinked to the samples, institutional review board review and approval are required and explicit consent likely would be needed.

It is important to raise the question of whether the controversy over the need for consent for use of residual blood spots places the highly successful population-based newborn-screening program at risk. I believe that newborn screening should be mandatory and should not require informed consent. The potential benefit to every newborn justifies this approach.

The critical issue is to safeguard the benefit to newborns of early detection of life-threatening conditions and initiation of treatment that is made possible by newborn screening. Whether there is a need to obtain permission for storage of samples after testing should not affect the debate about whether informed consent is required for newborn-screening programs in general. Discussion of the ability to opt in or out of storage of residual specimens should not be so frightening or confusing as to increase the likelihood that families will opt out of newborn screening for their babies.

Newborn Screening—Future Directions

Some states, with grants from the National Institutes of Health, are beginning to experiment with genomic testing to replace tandem mass spectrometry as the approach to newborn screening. Although this new technology is more expensive, it has the potential to replace a screening program with definitive diagnostic testing, dramatically expand the numbers of disorders tested, and significantly increase the number of incidental findings. A genetic-testing approach to newborn screening will require a reexamination of the basic principles of newborn screening and will create a great deal of controversy about the clinical utility and appropriateness of the information revealed to families. As the genomic information becomes more widely available, it is likely that many families will want to learn as much as they can about their child's genetic potential. Other families will want to protect themselves and their babies from the problems and self-fulfilling prophecies that such information might produce. I have serious concerns about the impact of universal genomic testing on future children and their families. I believe it will be impossible to limit testing to a small number of disorders for which treatment is available, as is done today. Other incidental findings of significance but not of imminent concern will be available and will likely be revealed to families with or without consent. Genomic testing of newborns will result in families learning many things they had not wished to know about their child and about themselves. A thoughtful ethical analysis of these issues will be important as the technology evolves.

BIOBANKING

In recent years, the creation of programs for storage of large numbers of biologic samples, (e.g. blood, body fluids, and tissues), linked with additional phenotypic, demographic, and personal health-related information, has become commonplace in academic research centers around the country. These biobanks, as they are called, are a research resource useful for exploring genetic hypotheses of various sorts. Some biobanks contain samples related to only one disease, whereas others may be broad based and representative of the entire population. Biobanks may contain hundreds or thousands or even hundreds of thousands of samples. State storage programs for research with residual blood spots from newborn screening are examples of population-based biobanking. Investigators associated with the state health department or with the academic center that create the biobank and other investigators not associated with that institution may study samples and linked information. Large information technology infrastructures are often associated with these biobanks in order to increase the potential to explore complex questions with very large data sets. Studies can measure genomic information or other biomarkers from stored specimens, and link that data to disease diagnoses, physical traits, or other demographic information available from the subjects.

The practice of biobanking raises many ethical questions and concerns. Can the privacy of subjects be adequately protected? What type of consent process is needed? May specimens from children who cannot consent for themselves be included in such banks? In addition, there has been a great deal of debate about the circumstances under which research findings should be revealed to subjects.

Biobanks promise subjects that their privacy will be preserved and protected. However, even when explicit identifiers such as name, address, and social security number are separated from the samples, it is possible in many instances to identify the subject by examining genomic markers or other demographic information. Since each person's genome is unique, if that person's genetic information was available on any other database that includes identifiers, it would be easy to discover the individual with virtual certainty. It is estimated that examining only 100 DNA fragments is needed to uniquely identify an individual with very high likelihood. Since currently there are very few genetic databases, the actual risk of a de-identified sample being used to identify an individual is very small. But the number of genomic databases is increasing. Using genomic information from biobank samples to identify individuals would require both significant effort and malicious and unethical motivation. Although most critical observers of the practice of biobanking are concerned about the possibility of using a biologic sample to identify an individual, demographic information is even more likely to be used to identify a specific person. The combination of date of birth, gender, and a five-digit zip code can identify over 50% of those living in the United States. These three data elements, combined with readily available databases like voter registration lists, can be used to easily identify individual subjects who are participants in a biobank.

Although the risks of breaches of privacy in biobanking and the revealing of confidential information about individuals is very small, I believe biobanks must take these risks into consideration in developing strategies both for determining what data are collected and for how the information is protected. Individual research scientists should also be held accountable for their actions. Substantial penalties should exist for researchers who do not abide by their commitment to keep information private and who unethically attempt to re-identify samples.

Biobank Institutional Review Boards

Biobanks should have review boards whose responsibility is to assure best practices in data management, and the protection of the anonymity of subjects. These boards should review the quality of research proposals that will utilize bank samples and data. Review boards should also develop and administer written agreements with investigators that clearly describe the responsibilities of investigators to protect subjects' anonymity. Investigators should be mandated to promise to use the samples only to perform the experiments that are approved by the biobank, and to generate no additional data from these samples. Such agreements (often called data-use agreements) should require the signature of the investigator and a senior administrative official at the investigator's institution. Data-use agreements acknowledge the institution's responsibility to supervise the ethical conduct of the investigator and to hold the investigator accountable if breaches of that responsibility occur.

Biobank—Informed Consent

The approach to informed consent for participation in a biobank is another controversial aspect of this type of research. Biobanks are conceived as repositories for samples and data that allow scientists to ask many research questions; some not even conceived when the samples were collected. Some biobanks relate exclusively to one type of disease, such as diabetes, cancer, heart disease, or autism. Other biobanks are more general in their orientation, encouraging exploratory research to reveal links between genetic and other biologic markers and disease. Potential participants in a biobank are often asked to give blanket consent to allow the biobank to perform any scientifically sound research using the samples over a very long period of time, perhaps forever. Some consent forms allow subjects to choose from a list of research areas in which they agree their samples may be utilized, whereas other consents do not provide any limits on sample use. Subjects are asked to trust the judgment of the managers of the bank, often a prestigious academic medical center or university, to provide appropriate stewardship. Subjects need to be assured that the samples and data will be used in a manner that develops important new knowledge to allow for better understanding of prevention and treatment of disease.

Some critics have argued that blanket consent is inappropriate, and that subjects should be recontacted in order to provide consent to participate in any new research that was not anticipated when the subject was first enrolled. Some biobanks have created sophisticated technologies to link subjects with the bank and enable continued dialogue about specific research project involvement. Although this appears to be working well for a small number of banks, most banks are not providing that level of interaction with participants. It seems reasonable that participants should be allowed to provide blanket permission for a very broad range of research studies upon enrollment in the biobank as long as the informed consent process is clear and explicit on this point. However, I believe that every biobank should develop a community advisory board, whose responsibility is to review each proposed research study in order to assure that the goals and objectives of the study are consistent with the general interests of the community from which the subjects where recruited. The community advisory board is not meant to provide scientific review, but rather it provides a voice to interact with the managers of the biobank to represent those who have given blanket consent and to assure that the research meets the intended goals and objectives of the biobank. This process also shows respect for the cultural and religious norms of the community.

Subjects are often told—and informed consent-forms document—that participants will receive no direct benefit from participating in a biobank, but that their enrollment may help others in the future. Participating in a biobank is an altruistic act for the sake of science and for the possible benefit of future patients. Nevertheless, biobank participants, like many other research subjects, are often confused about whether their participation may result in personal benefit. Participants are also naïve to the potential for biologic samples to be used for lucrative discoveries that result in considerable revenue for scientists and sponsoring institutions. Informed consent documents often note that there will be no compensation to subjects, but do not explain that samples may be used to develop financially profitable discoveries.

All these concerns about the informed-consent process demand that biobanks develop and institutional review boards approve informed-consent documents that are clear and comprehensive, dealing with each of the issues raised in this discussion. Recent work on interactive multimedia informed-consent tools that allow subjects to have questions answered and assess participant understanding of the research are a promising approach to obtaining informed-consent in biobanking.

Many biobanks wish to enroll children, raising additional questions about informed consent. Chapter 10 on research ethics will provide a more in-depth examination of the issue of informed consent for children who participate in research, but there are several issues concerning consent that are specific to biobanking. Should parents be permitted to enroll their children's samples and data in biobanks? Should biobanks be required to obtain the assent of a child to participate, either when they are first enrolled or when they become old enough? Should the informed consent of adolescents be required for continuing use of their samples and data in a biobank?

It seems reasonable for parents to be permitted to enroll their children's samples and data in biobanks and to provide permission for the use of samples to enhance scientific knowledge without direct benefit to the child. Although we have reviewed the risks of participation in biobanks, in general, those risks are minimal when biobanks act responsibly to protect the privacy of participants. The importance of exploratory genetic studies in childhood diseases, the low risk associated with participation in biobanks, and the general acceptance of parents as the appropriate surrogates for decisions on behalf of children makes obtaining parental permission for enrolling children in biobanks a reasonable and appropriate approach. It also seems reasonable to give the child the opportunity to assent to being part of these studies when he or she becomes sufficiently mature. The child's refusal to assent should be binding on the biobank, and no further studies on his or her sample should be permitted. Similarly, adolescents when they acquire the capacity to provide informed consent should be offered the opportunity to continue participation in the biobank or to have their samples destroyed based on refusal of continued participation.

Years after enrollment, it is possible that the biobank will be unable to find the child or adolescent to ask for permission to continue to use their specimens and data. Some commentators argue that without the explicit assent of the child or consent of the adolescent when he or she comes of age, the biobank should no longer be permitted to use the samples and data in any research studies. Although this is a justifiable argument in longitudinal research studies, in this case, where there is no ongoing contact with the research subject, risks are minimal, privacy is adequately protected, and due diligence has been done to search for the young person, I believe the biobank should be permitted to continue to use the samples and data while they periodically seek to determine the whereabouts of the person. Such policies should be explicitly mentioned in the informed consent process. These approaches should be reviewed periodically by the community advisory board and changes considered as the biobank continues to enroll subjects and evolve its practices.

Biobank—Revealing Research Findings

Individuals who participate in biobanks are informed that it is unlikely that they will derive any direct benefit from participation. But are there any obligations on the part of researchers or biobanks to return research results or incidental findings to individual participants if findings reveal information that could impact directly on the health or well-being of the subject or his or her family? Some biobanks receive truly anonymized samples with minimal data sets that make it virtually impossible to re-identify subjects. Most biobanks have de-identified coded samples with the capacity to re-identify a subject if necessary. At a minimum, biobanks and their associated investigators must address the question of return of research results and incidental findings. There should be explicit policies that articulate the bank's view of these obligations, and informed consent documents that make these policies clear to the participants. Participants should be informed whether the biobank will only return research results and incidental findings with their permission or whether the biobank intends to return all findings that meet certain health-related criteria.

I believe that participants, years after they checked off a box on an informed-consent document stating their preference for return of research results that had personal health-related importance, are likely to forget which box they checked or even what the various options were. Regardless of the prior choice, it is likely that they will assume that if an investigator has found meaningful information of importance to their personal health or the health and well-being of their family, that they would be informed. It is of note that many research subjects assume, often incorrectly, that researchers, like their physicians, are obligated by beneficence to behave in a manner that maximizes their interests; thus, they assume that important health-related findings will be revealed to them. Silence on the part of the research investigator is assumed by the participant to be an indication that there are no findings of concern.

At first glance, communicating research results that may have direct relevance to the health and well-being of the subject or his family may seem like a significant benefit to the participant. However, return of results can be associated with significant risks such as anxiety, depression, need and expense for confirmation and follow-up, and negative impact on other family members. To minimize the possibility of inflicting unnecessary harm on a subject by revealing a research result or incidental finding, the biobank must assure that the measured sample actually belongs to the purported individual and that the findings are analytically valid and consistent with the quality assurance standards of a certified clinical laboratory. This may sometimes require confirmatory testing in another laboratory.

The criteria for which research results will be returned also needs to be clarified. I believe that those results that have the potential for direct benefit to the subject should be revealed. Direct benefit can include genetic information or other findings that have important health implications for the individual or that can be used in reproductive decision-making to prevent or ameliorate a serious condition in a potential offspring. Some believe that only "actionable" findings should be returned, but the definition of *actionable* is controversial. *Actionable* can mean the ability to prevent or ameliorate a disease, but it can also include the ability to seek help in coping with or preparing for disease onset. When children are the subjects for whom results are available and there is no ability to directly intervene to prevent or ameliorate the disease, a discussion about return of results with their parents is needed. Assisting parents to deal with the information and determine when such information should be shared with their child (as discussed in the section on testing of children for adult onset disease) is warranted. Some might argue that if the information has no direct benefit to the child, it should not be revealed. But like the problem of revealing the results of secondary conditions in newborn screening, it is usually most appropriate to reveal the findings to the parents and counsel them about the implications.

Re-identifying the participant may not be difficult if there is a coded database, but finding the person may be more difficult if they have moved or relocated out of the area. There are many ways to find an individual, and diligent efforts should be undertaken. Finally, the actual revealing of results must be accomplished in a sensitive and professional manner.

Knowledgeable clinicians should be involved in this aspect of the process. Clinicians should be able to explain the findings and offer counsel about the genetic and reproductive implications of the information and make recommendations for needed follow-up.

Many of the early recommendations about withholding research results and incidental findings from subjects were based on the belief that researchers have no obligation to share results with participants. Paternalistic views that revealing the information would harm participants prevailed. Empirical data reveal that the vast majority of people expect to be informed about important information of personal or family relevance and that, with some support, they can readily cope with the implications of this information. Contemporary researchers need to understand that research subjects often conflate the roles of clinicians and researchers, and assume that all those people in white coats who are associated with academic medical centers and universities are motivated by having their best interests at heart. Ethical behavior in this circumstance should be motivated by an understanding of what the reasonable person would wish to know. Informing should be done respectfully, with sensitivity to the complexity and potential importance of the information.

WHOLE GENOME OR EXOME SEQUENCING

Whole genome testing for children with unusual and hard-to-diagnose diseases has become a part of pediatric practice in many academic medical centers. This testing is now recommended for children who have signs or symptoms that suggest a genetic disorder but for whom the known disease gene does not contain any mutation. Whole genome testing is also recommended for patients with serious, multisystem disorders that appear to be unique and might be caused by a genetic defect. Although this testing began and continues in many sites as a research study, some places are creating clinical programs available to test any patient whose sample is referred for analysis. As the sequencing technology becomes easier, information systems more robust, and the cost decreases, it has become attractive to consider examining DNA in the entire genome (or in the smaller fraction of the genome that constitutes the active coding regions, called the exome), to look for mutations that have the potential to be linked to the presenting phenotype of the patient. Testing is most often done on the patient as well as the parents to define the origin of the mutation and to inform the parents of their status as a carrier.

In a recent report, exome sequencing from 750 clinical patients were examined over a period of less than two years, by a clinically certified genetics laboratory, yielding a "diagnostic rate" of about 25% for unrelated metabolic disorders not previously suspected. Predictions are that this rate will increase as the techniques are enhanced and the numbers of known mutations related to various diseases increase. A major challenge at the present time is interpreting the data and determining which of the mutations are actually pathogenic and related to the clinical findings of the patient. In addition, the identification of a gene mutation plays little role in most cases in the clinical care and outcome for that patient. Such information may provide some solace to the family about the cause of the disorder, and if the findings show that a parent of the child carries the mutation, it can affect future reproductive decisions.

Whole genome or exome testing can increase clarity of diagnosis or causation in some cases, but the problem of incidental findings is immense. Whole genome or exome testing represents the first medical test that is guaranteed to produce abnormal findings in all who are tested. In the report cited earlier, there were more deleterious mutations found that were unrelated to the disease phenotype than mutations related to the disease. This creates extraordinary ethical concerns about whether to reveal incidental findings not related to the disease. The American College of Medical Genetics has provided some recommendations to researchers and clinicians for revealing incidental findings in whole genome sequencing, but this does not solve the ethical problems. The College recommends that certain health-related findings in whole exome testing are so important that laboratories have an ethical obligation to inform the patients or families of positive results regardless of whether they wish such information. Since the laboratory rarely has information about the clinical context of the testing, it is hard to generalize that in every instance it is in the interest of the patient/family to have this information.

Mr. and Mrs. Brandon, the parents of a two-year-old boy, George, in Case 3, were faced with great anxiety about their son's unexplained developmental delay. They were offered and consented to whole exome testing to help elucidate the cause of George's undiagnosed disorder. Although the genetic testing did not reveal any pathogenic mutations related to the disorder, incidental findings revealed that George had genetic mutations that dramatically increased his risk for breast cancer and Alzheimer's disease later in life. The parents reacted with great anxiety about George's future, and about the possibility that they themselves, as well as other family members, might be at increased risk for these disorders.

Many investigators and clinicians are not revealing incidental findings to families in a desire to protect them from confusing information of uncertain value. Some are counseling families about the existence of such information and allowing them to decide whether and how much they want to know. As with most new technological advances, the predictions of benefits and risks are initially exaggerated. There are some clinical and research programs that are experimenting with sophisticated, interactive websites that can inform subjects and their families about test results and incidental findings, and provide needed information. These types of programs will help to create best practices in this field, but there is still a great deal of work needed to clarify what information should be revealed and by what methodology. Ultimately, encouraging the patient—if he or she has the capacity to participate in the decision—and the family to become informed before consenting about what will be revealed by genomic testing and providing in-depth counseling about the meaning of the information will likely become standard practice and the most ethically reasonable approach.

I believe that, in the future, research using whole exome testing may result in many important findings about disease causation and prognosis, and may help create hypotheses about treatment interventions for genetic diseases. At present, it seems premature to make these tests widely available in the clinical domain. The lack of actionable findings related to the primary clinical question of concern and the large number of incidental findings justifies skepticism about the broad diffusion of this new technology into clinical care. If centers wish to pursue clinical application of exome testing, it is imperative that the informed consent process be comprehensive and clear. Families should be helped to make decisions about this testing without undue optimism about the clinical utility of the data, and with the understanding that they may learn genetic information that they did not wish to know about their child, themselves, and their family.

Whole genome sequencing has also had an impact on predictive genetic testing. Genetic entrepreneurs are marketing direct-to-consumer predictive genomic testing for such common chronic illnesses as cardiovascular disease, diabetes, and cancer, as well as testing for predispositions to behavioral risk factors such as those associated with obesity, addiction, and alcoholism. Many behavioral disorders have their origins in childhood, and anyone can submit the necessary biologic sample, generally saliva, and obtain the genetic results for a fee. There has been a great deal of criticism of this approach to genetic testing because of the lack of regulation of the quality of the laboratories and the questionable validity, reproducibility, and utility of the findings. In addition, there is concern for individuals to actively engage in destructive behaviors if they believe they have little genetic risk of illness or, alternatively, if they believe they are so predisposed to illness that nothing they can do will affect the outcome. The potential for harm to individuals is great if these private laboratories and genetic testing programs are not more carefully regulated to ensure the safety of the public.

FINAL THOUGHTS

Genetic testing and screening are becoming a more important part of clinical practice, and will undoubtedly provide many insights into disease risk, diagnosis, prevention, and treatment. Over time, the public will gain greater understanding of genetics and genomics, and common misperceptions about genetic determinism will decrease. Genetic information in general should be considered special in the sense that such information is relevant not only to the individual patient but also to his or her close relatives, and because the misuse of genetic information can be used to stigmatize or discriminate against individuals and their family members. This fact increases the complexity of the informed consent process for testing and the obligation of patient and clinician to consider whether to reveal relevant information to family members.

The increasing likelihood that whole genome testing will be used for clinical purposes and newborn screening presents serious concerns about revealing the incidental findings that will be generated in virtually every case. I believe we can develop reasonable approaches to these issues, but currently there is no consensus about what ought to be done. Parents need to be well counseled about the implications of genetic testing before consenting, and well-intentioned clinicians need to be aware of the foreseeable negative consequences of obtaining genetic information of little clinical utility.

It is likely that the impact of the genetic revolution in the next 50 years will be less positive than hoped for by scientists today, but with increased understanding about genetic information there will also be less anxiety and fear among the public than is currently predicted.

ADDITIONAL READINGS

American Academy of Pediatrics Committee on Bioethics, and Committee on Genetics, and the American College of Medical Genetics and Genomics Social,

Ethical and Legal Issues Committee. Ethical and policy issues in genetic testing and screening of children. *Pediatrics*, 2013; 131(3): 620–622.

Botkin JR, Goldenberg A, Rothwell E, et al. Retention and research use of residual newborn screening bloodspots. *Pediatrics* 2013; 131: 120–127.

Charlisse E, Caga-anan F, Smith L, et al. Testing children for adult-onset genetic diseases. *Pediatrics*, 2012; 129(1): 163–168.

Clayton EW. Genetic testing in children. *J Med Philos*, 1997; 22: 233–251.

Feero WG, Guttmacher AE, Collins FS, Genomic medicine—an updated primer. *N Engl J Med*, 2010; 362: 2001–2011.

Fleischman AR, Lin BK, Howse JL. A commentary on the President's Council on Bioethics report: The changing moral focus of newborn screening. *Genet Med*, 2009; 11: 507–509.

Green RC, Berg JS, Grody WW, et al. ACMG recommendations for reporting of incidental findings in clinical exome and genome sequencing. *Genet Med*, 2013; 15: 565–574.

Ross LF. Ethical and policy issues in pediatric genetics. *Am J Med Genet Part C: Semin Med Genet*, 2008; 148C(1): 1–7.

Soden, SE, Farrow EG, Saunders CJ, et al. "Genomic medicine: evolving science, evolving ethics." *Personal Med*, 2012; 9(5): 523–528.

Tarini BA, Tercyak KP, Wilfond BS. Children and predictive genomic testing: disease prevention, research protection, and our future. *J Pediat Psychol*, 2011; 36(10): 1113–1121.

Yang Y, Muzny DM, Reid JG, et al. Clinical whole-exome sequencing for the diagnosis of mendelian disorders. *N Engl J Med*, 2013; 369: 1502–1511.

CHAPTER 6
Ethical Issues at the End of Life

Caring for Gravely Ill Children

Case 1

Barbara Todd and her 4-year-old son, Michael, were playing soccer on a beautiful day in the backyard near their swimming pool. Barbara heard the phone ring and went to answer the call on the portable phone she had left in the kitchen. She returned in a few minutes to the horrifying sight of Michael floating face down in the pool. She screamed and jumped into the pool to pull Michael out. Michael's father, William, heard Barbara scream, called 911, and initiated resuscitative efforts. The ambulance came quickly and the emergency medical technicians intubated the child and brought him to the hospital. After four days in the hospital on a ventilator, with no signs of neurologic recovery, clinicians suspected that Michael was brain dead. Nurses and doctors talked to the Todds about hospital procedures for determining brain death and about the various options for organ donation. Barbara and William were confused and concerned. They were reluctant to accept that Michael might be dead. They hoped he might recover, and they did not wish to give up hope.

Case 2

Mohamed Gupta is a 10-year-old boy with a malignant brain tumor. He was operated on by Dr. Michael Porter, the chief of neurosurgery at the local children's hospital who found a very invasive tumor that was impossible to fully remove. Dr. Henry Baumgartner, the pediatric oncologist, initiated chemotherapy but shared his pessimistic outlook with Mohamed's parents, Charles and Portia. The Guptas were devastated by the news that Mohamed would likely die from this malignancy, but requested that all the doctors and nurses tell the boy that his tumor was completely removed and that he would be fine after some additional treatments. Dr. Baumgartner was reluctant to agree to their request, but they insisted. One of the pediatric nurse practitioners on the oncology service told the Guptas that she would not lie to Mohamed. They asked that she not be involved in Mohamed's care. Dr. Baumgartner acceded to their wishes, citing the recent information he received from the hospital administration about the importance of family-centered care and respect for parents' views and values. He assigned a senior fellow to be in charge of Mohamed's care and rarely returned to the bedside.

Each year in the United States about 2.5 million people die. Only 44,000 of these deaths occur in children. A bit more than half of pediatric deaths occur during the first year of life, primarily due to the consequences of prematurity, or birth with a congenital abnormality, or a serious genetic or metabolic disorder. As children get older, the main causes of death are accidents, cancer, and heart disease. Most children who are seriously, critically, or terminally ill are cared for in children's hospitals by highly trained pediatric subspecialists. And most pediatric deaths occur in these settings.

Medical care that is likely to achieve cure or to restore a seriously ill child to health and normal function, such as antibiotics for meningitis, insulin for diabetes, or surgery to set a fractured bone, rarely poses an ethical dilemma. In these instances, parental religious beliefs, economic factors, or the child and family's ability to adjust to the requirements of the treatment regimen will occasionally raise questions or problems, but clinicians generally can pursue a clear and uncontroversial course of treatment that will return the child to health. When parents choose to refuse clearly beneficial and efficacious treatment, legal mechanisms exist for society, represented by the state, to assure the provision of such treatments.

Often, however, when children are gravely ill, proposed treatments may not easily be classified as likely to achieve cure or restore health and normal function. Rather than being clearly beneficial or efficacious, treatments may be marginally beneficial and of uncertain efficacy. In order to decrease controversy and conflict, and to facilitate decision-making in such cases, pediatric practitioners and children's hospitals have developed policies and practices that embrace what is called patient- and family-centered care. This approach recognizes that the patient and family are integral partners with the healthcare team. Patients, regardless of age, are respected and involved in decisions about their care consistent with their cognitive ability and developmental level. Families are respected as playing a vital role in ensuring the health and well-being of children. The term *family* is broadly defined and may encompass a multiplicity of parenting and multigenerational relationships. Children's hospitals and pediatricians have accepted the core principles of family-centered care including sharing information openly and honestly with patients and families; fostering collaboration of children and parents as collaborators in all decisions that affect the child; and incorporating the family's racial, ethnic, religious, and cultural values and preferences into planning for the child's care.

Family-centered care promotes effective communication between clinicians and families and encourages a respectful relationship to decrease the likelihood of conflict or disagreement. However, despite best intentions, legitimate disagreements may occur between doctors, or between doctor, patient, and family about how best to proceed with the care of a seriously ill or dying child. The doctor or the family may wish to provide all available treatments regardless of how marginal the benefit. As the child's prognosis worsens, and uncertainty about outcome decreases, a consensus about the overall goals of care and the desirability of specific interventions must be developed. Continued focus solely on treatment can deflect the child and the family from integrating the reality of the impending death, and can increase the child's suffering.

Adults with the capacity to make healthcare decisions for themselves are generally respected as autonomous, and are given the unfettered authority to accept or refuse any offered treatments. Clinicians and family members may believe that an autonomous adult's decision to accept or refuse a treatment is not in his or her own interest, but respect for that person's right to make the choice obligates the clinician to proceed as requested by the patient. However, the concept of respect for autonomy only invokes a negative right, the right to refuse an intervention. It is not a positive right, the right to demand a treatment that is not being offered.

For children who are incapable of making informed choices, parents or guardians play the role of surrogate decision-maker. Older children who have the capacity to participate in decision-making about their own care need to be integrated into this process in a manner consistent with their cognitive ability and developmental level. Children should be informed about the nature of their condition, the proposed treatment plan, and the expected outcome in understandable terms appropriate to their developmental levels.

Some adolescents should be given the autonomous right to make choices for themselves, regardless of parental wishes; but for the vast majority of children, parents will be the healthcare decision-makers. The deference to parental choice is consistent with family-centered care; it promotes and respects the value of family integrity, ensures the identification of a decision-maker, and acknowledges the legitimate role parents play in shaping their children's lives. However, parents are not autonomous decision-makers for their children. Parents are charged with the responsibility of asking what best promotes the child's interest. Parents may not refuse clearly beneficial medical treatments, without which the child is likely to suffer irrevocable harm. Physicians who care for children are given the responsibility to make independent assessments of the best interest of their patients, and to advocate for their patient when parents refuse known efficacious treatments. In addition, parents may not demand treatments for their child that are not medically indicated and, therefore, not offered by their child's physicians.

Some parents regard survival of their child in a debilitated condition as undesirable, and may resist treatments proposed by clinicians that are unlikely to fully restore their child's health and function. Other parents believe that life has value regardless of disability or handicap and will request treatments sometimes resisted by physicians. In determining the best interests of any child, the quality of the child's life following treatment is central to decision-making. Reasonable people may disagree about what the future quality of life will be and about what quality of life is worth sustaining. Parents can legitimately reject treatments that merely prolong the dying process, increase pain and suffering for their child, or will not be effective in enhancing the child's well- being. When clinicians offer treatments, or parents make best-interest choices about treatments, it is important to recognize possible biases about the burdens of living with illness and disability. It is helpful to consider the enormous adaptability of children and the range of possibilities and experiences reported by individuals who live with similar conditions.

When physicians and nurses, practicing in children's hospitals and large pediatric services in general hospitals are surveyed, they voice serious concerns of conscience about overtreating children in their care. The great majority of clinicians say that they sometimes feel that they are saving children who should not be saved, and that treatments that are offered to critically ill children are sometimes overly burdensome. Attending physicians surveyed are about 10 times as worried, and nurses are over 20 times as worried about saving children who should not be saved as they are about giving up on children too soon.

Studies of clinicians also reveal lack of knowledge about basic ethical guidelines for pediatric end-of-life care, including the definition of brain death, the implementation of organ donation after circulatory death, the distinction between withholding and withdrawing of treatment from gravely ill children, the withdrawal of medically provided nutrition and hydration in a terminally ill child, and provision of adequate pain management to a suffering child. Although there have been many consensus statements and published guidelines about each of these issues, clinicians often have individual views that differ significantly from practice guidelines. These broad differences in views and values, combined with the differing values and preferences of patients and families, create many conflicts and ethical dilemmas in the care of gravely ill children.

BRAIN DEATH IN CHILDREN

Brain death is the complete and irreversible cessation of all brain function including the brain stem, responsible for involuntary activity like breathing. This definition joins the more classic definition of death, the irreversible cessation of circulatory and respiratory function, as one of the two generally accepted definitions of death. The concept of brain death was created in the 1960s as a social construct, developed in response to the desire to procure organs for transplantation from dying patients before circulatory collapse made the organs not viable. Guidelines for the clinical determination of the complete cessation of all brain function in adults were developed in the 1960s and 1970s, and states adopted laws accepting brain death as legal death in order to permit the transplantation of organs from adults who were brain dead and being sustained on ventilators (Uniform Anatomical Gift Act). There was limited experience and little systematic evidence about determining brain death in pediatric patients, but guidelines for children were first widely accepted and published in the late 1980s. Although the guidelines were generally accepted for older children, there remained concern that infants less than a year of age might require special confirmatory testing, and that, because of brain development and plasticity, determination of brain death might not be possible in neonates.

Recently, the American Academy of Pediatrics published updated guidelines for determining brain death in pediatric patients. These guidelines apply to all children including neonates and infants. A child with a known irreversible cause of coma is determined to be brain dead when there is complete absence of all neurologic function. All physiologic disturbances including hypotension, hypothermia, and metabolic abnormalities must be corrected prior to the determination. All drugs that might affect the neurologic examination, such as sedatives, analgesics, anticonvulsants, and neuromuscular blocking agents, must be discontinued and a reasonable time must transpire so that the drugs are no longer active in the body. Two separate examinations are required including an apnea test in each instance, and an observation period between tests of 12–24 hours, depending on the age of the child. Ancillary laboratory and imaging studies are not required unless the clinical testing cannot be performed adequately. Death is declared after the second confirmatory test is completed.

These guidelines have clarified the necessary procedures to determine that a child is brain dead, but they have not addressed some continuing ethical concerns. Patients who meet the medical criteria for brain death actually continue to have many physiologically significant brain functions, including hormonal regulation and temperature control. These patients have lost all neurologic function, are in coma, and are not able to breath, but they have not suffered "complete and irreversible cessation of all brain function," as required by law. This distinction between the definition of brain death and biologic reality is theoretically important but it has not affected public consensus or public policy about the utility of brain death as a legal definition of death. This is important because utilizing the brain death criteria to determine death supports the public consensus that permits vital organ removal for transplantation only from patients who have already died. Our society strongly holds that organ removal per se should not cause the death of the patient.

The fact that brain dead individuals can maintain hormonal regulation and temperature control, and ventilators can maintain oxygenation and cardiac function make those who are brain dead look like living patients who are asleep or in coma. This apparent contradiction adds to the confusion and sense of denial most parents experience when facing the death of their child. This often affects the response of parents who have been told that their child is brain dead. In Case 1 in this chapter, the Todds sat by the bedside of their son, Michael, holding his hand while the doctors discussed the process for determining brain death. Michael looked asleep; he didn't look dead. He was warm and pink, his chest moved up and down, and the monitors showed that his pulse and blood pressure were normal. The healthcare professionals caring for Michael were empathic about the turmoil the Todds were experiencing. They explained that first the neurologist, and then, 12 hours later, the intensive care attending physician would perform a complete neurologic assessment of Michael, including a test of his ability to breath without ventilatory support (an apnea test). If both examinations confirmed the absence of brain function, Michael would be declared dead and removed from the respirator. The family would be given a bit of time to accept this plan; but after the patient is declared brain dead, hospital policy required only a "reasonable accommodation" to the family's religious or personal views about removing the patient from the ventilator. In almost every state, doctors do not need permission from the family to perform the examinations nor to withdraw the ventilator if brain death is confirmed.

The language used to refer to brain dead patients by clinicians, family, friends, and the general public adds to the confusion about brain death. Out of respect for the dead and for their family, we do not refer to brain dead patients as cadavers or corpses, but this adds to the perception that the loved one is not dead, merely very sick. The media often reports that the family "decided" to withdraw the ventilator and allow the child to die after the determination that the patient was brain dead. Clinicians sometimes make an error and ask permission from a family to remove the respirator from a patient who has been declared brain dead, confusing the approach to asking permission to withdraw a respirator from a child who is not dead but critically and irreversibly ill with the protocol for a child who is brain dead. Requesting permission implies choice. Although families should be informed that their child has died and that the respirator will be removed, they should be given a brief period of time to adapt to that reality, and they may wish to be present when the child is removed from the machine.

Although flawed in its conceptual basis, because brain death does not represent the complete cessation of all brain function, the concept of brain death remains an important contributor to societal good. Although the determination of brain death may not be consistent with the complete and irreversible cessation of all brain functions, it does define a condition of severe and irreversible coma with lack of all neurologic function. For individuals who are brain dead, continued treatment has no potential to reverse profound brain dysfunction or to provide any hope for future benefit; these individuals are clearly appropriate candidates for vital organ donation.

At the heart of the current controversy inside the ethics community about the definition of brain death is the belief by some that a potential organ donor should not need to be declared dead before vital organs may be removed for transplantation. These commentators believe that the Uniform Anatomical Gift Act should be modified to permit organs to be removed from persons who are not yet dead. Although I am very sympathetic to this view and believe that families should be permitted to donate their loved one's vital organs before they have died, as part of the process of withdrawing treatment at the end of life, I am very concerned that all of this discussion will escalate to the level of creating fear and confusion among the public that might result in lessening the supply of transplantable organs for children in need. Mistrust of the motives of the medical profession combined with a strongly held societal belief that donating organs should not be the immediate cause of death could result in families not permitting organ donation from their loved ones who have actually been declared dead.

ORGAN DONATION AFTER CIRCULATORY DEATH

Hundreds of children are on transplant lists awaiting the availability of a major organ, and many die each year while waiting. As transplantation of hearts, lungs, livers, and kidneys have been shown to be efficacious treatments for many serious diseases affecting children, there is an increasing need for pediatric transplantable organs, yet there are few brain dead pediatric patients who are suitable donors. There are, however, some families who wish to withdraw treatment to allow their children to die and would be willing to donate vital organs to help save the lives of other children. Since patients must be dead before vital organs may be removed, a relatively new program for obtaining organs has been developed—namely, organ donation after circulatory death. This approach to organ harvesting utilizes the circulatory definition of death. Organs are retrieved from patients after the planned withdrawal of life-sustaining treatment and declaration of death based on cessation of circulatory function. Waiting periods after stopping the respirator of as little as 75 seconds to as long as five minutes have been used before death is declared and organ retrieval initiated. The cessation of circulatory function is said to be permanent, but not irreversible. It is permanent because circulation will not start on its own or as a result of cardiopulmonary resuscitation, since as a part of the decision to withdraw life-sustaining treatment, the parents or guardian previously decided to forego all life-sustaining treatment including cardiopulmonary resuscitation. Once the patient is declared dead, respiratory support and circulation are restored in order to preserve vital organs for harvesting.

There are two conceptual criticisms of this highly controversial approach to retrieving vital organs. First, irreversibility of cessation of circulatory function has been viewed as a necessary criterion for the declaration of death using the circulatory criterion. With this approach, irreversibility is replaced by permanence through the mechanism of the do-not-resuscitate order that accompanies the planned withdrawal of treatment. Cessation of circulatory function is clearly reversible in these patients and is restarted after the declaration of death. This process seems somewhat disingenuous; with one commentator calling these organ donors "kinda dead," rather than really dead. The second criticism is that substituting permanence for irreversibility in the definition of death makes the definition contingent on the intent of the decision-makers rather than the intrinsic condition of the patient. Although some commentators find nothing wrong with intent of the decision-makers as sufficient to warrant this approach, I believe that the protocols for organ donation after circulatory death are somewhat hypocritical and pay only lip service to the definition of circulatory death.

In addition to conceptual criticisms, there are obvious conflicts of interest that must be considered. In contrast to donors declared brain dead, in donation after circulatory death, preparation for organ recovery begins before death is declared. This is necessary because vital organs might be damaged by decreased perfusion between the time of withdrawal of life support and recovery of the organs. Premortem interventions may include placing intravenous and arterial lines, administering anticoagulants such as heparin, and moving the patient to the operating room for withdrawal of life support. In addition, the fact that death occurs in the operating room separates the family from the child at the time of death. I believe these interventions prioritize the interests of the organ recipient over the interests of the donor and his or her family.

Present guidelines for organ donation after circulatory death take into consideration these criticisms and potential conflicts. Guidelines require that policies clearly separate the decision to withdraw life-sustaining treatment from the decision to donate the critically ill child's organs. Families are not approached about organ donation until after they have decided to withdraw life-sustaining treatment and allow their child to die. Premortem interventions require the consent of parent or guardian, and should not be painful or harmful to the patient. Parents are allowed to accompany their child to the doors of the operating room, but they may not be permitted inside the operating room where declaration of death will occur. Physicians responsible for withdrawal of treatment and declaration of death must be different from the team who will retrieve organs for transplantation.

Returning to our Case 1, when the neurologist formally assessed Michael, he suspected that he would find him to be brain dead, but some primitive corneal reflexes and attempts at breathing during the apnea test resulted in the conclusion that the patient was severely and irreversibly impaired but not brain dead. Confirmatory electroencephalograms during the next week revealed almost no electrical activity in the brain and repeat neurological exams revealed no improvement. Michael's parents, Barbara and William, became convinced that there was no hope that their son would recover. They asked the doctors to withdraw the ventilator and allow Michael to die. The critical-care specialists agreed and asked the Todds to speak with members of the organ procurement team to discuss the possibility of Michael becoming an organ donor. Although the Todds were willing to discuss the possibility of Michael becoming an organ donor, they were unwilling to subject him to the premortem procedures required by the organ donation after circulatory death protocol. And, they wanted him to be with at the time of death.

I am convinced that the practice of organ donation after circulatory death will force the field of transplantation and the society at large to address the question of whether an organ donor must be declared dead before organs may be retrieved. Families of a gravely ill child, who have decided to allow their loved one to die by having life support withdrawn can achieve some solace from these tragic circumstances by permitting organ donation. But these families must participate in stretching the boundaries of the accepted approach to declaring a patient dead after cessation of circulatory and respiratory function. Courageous and generous families may be willing to confront the need to develop new approaches for retrieval of vital organs before death is declared from patients who will inevitably die from withdrawal of treatment. This would reverse the dead-donor rule and require the Uniform Anatomical Death Act to be amended. It seems to me that this is the correct direction to take, since our present practices are open to serious criticism as being disingenuous and may jeopardize the laudable goal that they seek to support—increasing organ donation.

Is our society ready to address the need for organ donation, and is it willing to allow organ retrieval before irreversible cessation of all brain or circulatory function? I believe that our society is not ready to condone the fact that vital organ procurement could be a contributing factor to the death of a patient who is nonetheless inevitably dying. Until such a discussion results in a new societal consensus, our public policies and medical practices concerning organ transplantation will be hard to justify. Yet, as the need for vital organs continues to increase, it is hard to be critical of those who seek to encourage organ donation from families grieving for the loss of a cherished child.

WITHHOLDING VERSUS WITHDRAWAL OF TREATMENT

It has been recognized by healthcare professionals for decades that there is a significant psychological difference between stopping a treatment already in progress and not starting it in the first place. Withholding life-sustaining treatments is often felt to be an act of omission that permits death, whereas withdrawing treatments is more like an active intervention to hasten death. But, over the last 30 years, nationally prominent organizations and institutions like the American Medical Association, The Hastings Center, and the President's Commission for the Study of Ethical Problems in Medicine have provided guidelines for clinicians that clearly state there is no ethical distinction between withholding and withdrawing life-sustaining medical treatments. How do the guidelines justify this assertion that there is no ethical difference between stopping and not starting a medical treatment, and why do so many clinicians not accept these justifications?

The justification lies with balancing the obligation of physicians to offer medical treatments thought to be in the interests of a patient with the obligation to respect the right of patients and surrogates to reject treatments they do not believe to be in the patient's best interests. Decisions to forego life-sustaining treatments are so fundamental and important that they should never be made without considering the values and preferences of the involved patient and of the family when the patient does not have the capacity to participate in the decision. When a physician withholds or withdraws a treatment on the request of a patient or surrogate, the physician has fulfilled the obligation to offer appropriate medical treatment to the patient. The obligation to offer treatment does not include the obligation to impose treatment on an unwilling patient. In the case of a child, only if the physician can argue that the parent or guardian is making a decision that is clearly against the interest of the child may he or she seek court intervention to impose treatment. Since the earliest of such cases, courts have consistently upheld the right of competent patients and their surrogates to reject life-sustaining treatments.

So, it is surprising to learn that when pediatricians are surveyed, many do not agree that there is no ethical or legal distinction between withholding and withdrawing life-sustaining treatments. About half the pediatric oncologists surveyed believe there is an ethical difference between stopping and not starting a medical treatment. Withdrawing life-sustaining treatments already begun often feels psychologically more troubling than not starting a life-sustaining treatment. Physicians and nurses may be reluctant to withdraw treatments that will result in death because they feel that they become the agent causing the death, as might be the case in physician-assisted dying or euthanasia. When treatments are not initiated, clinicians generally think that their intention is to let the disease take its course, or to not prolong the dying process, with death the likely outcome of the decision. This approach is often more comfortable for clinicians and sometimes more acceptable to patients and surrogates. Physicians and nurses often feel more comfortable not starting a life-sustaining ventilator for respiratory failure, or dialysis for kidney failure, or antibiotics for an infection, than withdrawing these treatments after initiation.

Some commentators have argued that withdrawing a life-sustaining treatment after a time-limited trial of therapy during which time the effectiveness of the treatment can be assessed, may be "more ethical" than not initiating the treatment. I agree with this approach, but caution clinicians who might be reluctant to withdraw treatments that initiation of a questionable life-sustaining treatment is only acceptable if there will be the possibility to assess efficacy and withdraw the treatment after a short trial. When allowing death is the intended objective of withholding or withdrawing of a life-sustaining therapy, and a good process has been instituted to come to that conclusion, clinicians should be aware that there is no ethical or legal distinction between withholding or withdrawing.

MEDICALLY PROVIDED NUTRITION AND HYDRATION

Provision of food and water to sick and debilitated children is generally seen as an act of caring and compassion. Withholding medically provided food and water from elderly adults who are terminally ill is an accepted practice that has been utilized extensively to alleviate suffering and allow death. Should withholding or withdrawing of medically provided nutrition and hydration from gravely ill children with the intent of allowing death be permitted? Are such practices unacceptable and a form of dispassionate abandonment of vulnerable children?

Since the early 20th century, sick newborns and young children unable to eat have received nourishment through tubes inserted into their nose or mouth and gently advanced into the stomach. Intravenous infusions were also used to administer fluids containing electrolytes and glucose with a limited capacity to provide calories and no ability to provide proteins. In the late 1960s, a breakthrough, initially called hyperalimentation, was introduced to reverse the weight loss and inability to nourish newborns and infants with serious congenital abnormalities and bowel diseases that required surgical intervention. This new approach used intravenous infusions to optimize nutrition by providing not only electrolytes and high concentrations of glucose, but also proteins, fats, vitamins, and trace elements. Prior to this intravenous nutrition, infants often died of inanition and malnutrition after successful surgery of a correctable problem. Today, the vast majority of infants in neonatal intensive care and pediatric critical care units are nourished with medically provided feeding tubes or intravenous lines. Under what circumstances, if any, would it be ethically acceptable to withdraw or withhold this medically provided nutrition and hydration from gravely ill children to allow their death?

Many clinicians who care for children are emotionally uncomfortable with forgoing medically provided nutrition and hydration for their patients, and deem the practice unethical. Without question, intentionally depriving a healthy child of food and water is a monstrous act that will cause suffering and could inevitably result in death. But, the medical provision of nutrition and hydration for a gravely ill child may not prolong life, may cause significant pain and suffering, and may be inconsistent with the best interest of that child. Provision of intravenous nutrition and hydration can cause serious problems of overhydration, development of edema, heart failure, and liver and kidney failure in gravely ill children. Provision of nutrition and hydration directly into the stomach may cause severe pain and discomfort in dying children. In such circumstances, the emotionally wrenching decision to withdraw feeding tubes or intravenous nutrition may be ethically acceptable and appropriate. In gravely ill children who have had medically provided nutrition and hydration withdrawn, discomfort is rare and can be alleviated with attention to symptom management.

There is great symbolic significance in providing food to children, and caregivers understandably may experience psychological distress when they withhold nutrition and hydration. But well-meaning clinicians should not impose inappropriate ethical absolutes, and gravely ill and dying children should never be deprived of the option of having burdensome life-sustaining treatments withdrawn to allow a comfortable death.

PAIN MANAGEMENT AT THE END OF LIFE

Over the last decade, clinicians have been increasingly aware of the obligation to alleviate pain and suffering in critically and chronically ill children. Patient-rated pain scales are assessed routinely in hospitalized patients and analgesics and anesthetics are used more frequently for children in pain and during procedures. Of course, neonates and young infants cannot report their pain, but increased heart rate, crying, and agitation can be interpreted as signs of pain requiring treatment. Yet, clinicians report that they believe a significant number of pediatric patients are undermedicated for pain. These same clinicians believe that a major reason that children receive inadequate pain medication is the fear of hastening death. Such fear is misplaced on clinical, ethical, and legal grounds.

Data show that respiratory depression resulting in death is extremely rare in children receiving narcotic medications for pain. Even patients with altered mental status, disordered control of respiration, and abnormal renal and hepatic function can receive opioids safely if the drugs are administered gradually and titrated to effect. Neonatologists, critical-care physicians, oncologists, and experts in pain management have developed various multidrug regimens to deal with pain and the anxiety associated with fear of pain in children. Parents and clinicians observing children may sometimes underestimate the need for pain medication in a child who does not complain or becomes agitated when experiencing substantial pain. Experienced clinicians can titrate medications to alleviate even minor symptoms and the observed changes in vital signs, such as heart rate and blood pressure, which can be associated with pain.

But can we justify utilizing increasing levels of pain medications that might depress respirations or hasten death in a gravely ill patient? The first ethical justification of this practice is the obligation of physicians to alleviate pain and suffering. When patients are gravely ill and available treatments are not likely to result in cure or restoration of function, the focus of care must be on symptom management. Relief from pain and suffering is important for the child, and is often essential at the end of life.

A second ethical justification for the use of adequate pain management is the doctrine of "double effect." This doctrine comes primarily from Catholic teaching and is utilized to determine when an act that has both good and bad effects is permissible. Permissibility depends on whether the bad effect is intended and not merely foreseeable. If the bad effect is intended, it is not permissible; but if the bad effect is foreseeable but not intended, it is permissible. Intrinsically wrong acts, like killing, are not permitted. In the case of providing medication to alleviate pain and suffering for a gravely ill child that might hasten his or her death, the act itself is not intrinsically wrong, in fact it is laudable. The foreseeable bad effect, hastening death, is not the intended goal and is not necessary to achieve the intended goal of alleviating pain and suffering. The alleviation of pain is a sufficiently desirable goal to allow the bad effect, hastening death, to occur in some cases. Although most clinicians accept the doctrine of double effect and believe it is a good ethical justification for utilizing adequate pain management even if it may hasten death, they believe that hastening death is illegal. Adequate pain management at the end of life is not illegal; in fact, it has been called a constitutional right.

The Supreme Court of the United States in 1997 deliberated two cases associated with the right to assisted suicide. The Court concluded that states may prohibit physician assistance in dying, but no state may prohibit adequate palliative care, including pain relief, even if the medication hastens the death of the patient. The Court emphasized that a strong argument could be made for a constitutional right to "die with dignity," and this right requires the provision of sufficient medication to control pain, despite the risk that those drugs might cause the death of the patient.

Although pain management at the end of life for children is improving, all clinicians need to be educated in the most effective methods to prescribe and deliver the needed medications, and to be reassured that it is ethically and legally acceptable, in fact mandatory, to alleviate pain and suffering for all children at the end of life.

CHILDREN AS PARTICIPANTS IN PLANNING CARE

Although most children lack the capacity to make binding choices about their healthcare, the child's individual needs, interests, and perspectives must be the central focus of the decision. Clinicians should recognize that many health-related decisions permit participation of even very young children. The role of a child in planning care is less determined by chronologic age than by developmental and personal capacity. Very young children often have a keen understanding of their clinical situation; the importance of tests and treatments; and the associated burdens of hospital visits, pain, discomfort, and limitation of activity. It is important to engage children in discussion of their perceptions of these burdens and to allow them to verbalize their feelings, choose methods to enhance their comfort, and permit them to control the situation as much as possible. At the same time, care must be taken not to mislead or deceive children about their degree of authority for choices about tests and treatments. Parents and clinicians should avoid asking for a child's permission if a negative answer would be unacceptable. If a procedure must be performed, honesty and respect for the child demands that he or she be offered a limited but feasible range of options. For example, the child might determine the order in which a needed bone marrow aspirate and spinal tap are performed, or decide which arm will be the site of an intravenous line.

As children become older and attain greater capacity, they should be involved more fully in planning their care. Older children and adolescents may have religious or other values that shape their responses to illness and treatment. Often children are able to articulate personal goals and views about their end-of-life care and even about their death. These perspectives should be elicited through a series of discussions and should be given great weight. There is no simple formula to determine whether or to what extent a child is capable of participating in planning for their care. Parents and clinicians must jointly decide how much input and authority to give a child for making choices about treatment decisions. They need to take into account not only the child's level of understanding and ability to anticipate future consequences of present actions, but also the gravity of the decision in question, the risks and benefits of the options, and the probability and severity of the burdens of the treatment.

Parents, like the Guptas in Case 2 in this chapter, who ask the doctors not to disclose the prognosis of a malignant brain tumor to their 10-year-old son, often wish to protect their children from knowledge about their illness, particularly as they become more ill near the end of life. Family-centered care argues that parents' views and values should be respected in all issues concerning their child. But does family-centered care require clinicians to comply with the request to not disclose information or even to lie to their patients? What should clinicians do when they are asked not to disclose important information to a child about diagnosis, prognosis, or impending death?

There are several myths and misconceptions that generally accompany parental requests for keeping important information from children. Parents often believe that their child doesn't know much about his illness and has little interest in knowing more, that it is not hard to keep secrets from a child, and that the child does not have the capacity to understand the complexity of the situation. Also parents fear that disclosure will elevate the child's anxiety and compromise coping, and they wish to maintain an atmosphere of optimism and hope. Each of these beliefs is fraught with problems.

It is very hard to keep secrets from children. Even young children know they are ill, and they worry about what that means for their future. Children who have not been given the opportunity to understand their illness exhibit significantly greater distress, more internalization of problems, and increased symptoms of depression. Children often wish to please their parents and to protect them. They go along with their parents' wishes. When parents do not want them to know much about their illness, they ask few questions and accept the isolation and confusion of not knowing. Many studies have shown that honest and sensitive disclosure of illness status to children decreases anxiety, increases self-esteem, promotes a sense of mastery, and encourages adherence to medical regimens.

Clinicians who agree to keep important information from their patients, like Dr. Baumgartner in our case, generally decrease their interactions with the child because they fear they will divulge something they should not. This often causes the child to distrust professionals and to wonder why no one is talking to him. Conspiracies of silence can be very detrimental to both clinicians and patients. Clinicians become distressed about not fulfilling their obligations to their patient, and patients develop fantasies about their illnesses, often believing that it must be pretty awful if no one wants to talk about it. Respect for the child and the known negative consequences of nondisclosure-of-illness status obligate clinicians to ensure that their patient receives an appropriate level of information about his or her illness.

Sharing information with a child who is gravely ill and learning about a child's hopes and fears can give parents and clinicians valuable insights into what the illness means to the child, how he or she is coping, and what is important to them as individuals. In order to facilitate disclosure of information to children, I believe clinicians should validate the parents' views and express understanding of their values, confirming that there are some parents who believe children should not be told about their illness. But parents must be made aware of the negative consequences of not telling, and should be informed that the clinicians propose to develop an alliance with them to work together to inform the child. If parents insist on not allowing their child to be given any information about his or her illness, clinicians should inform the parents that they believe this is harmful to the child and that they will continue to try to convince the family to change their mind about this important issue. Minimally, clinicians should inform parents that they will not lie to the child and that all questions from the child will be answered truthfully, in a manner consistent with the child's developmental level. Disclosure-of-illness status should be seen as an incremental process. Taking cues from the child, information should be shared in small doses over time. All questions from the child should be answered honestly, remembering that children do not need long answers to short questions. If the disease progresses and the child is, in fact, dying, I believe he or she must be told and helped to cope with impending death. Families should not be permitted to allow their own grief and pain concerning their child's impending death to keep the child from learning the truth. Children, like adults, need time to prepare for their own death and want time to complete unfinished tasks and to say goodbye to those they love.

When cure or restoration of function is no longer possible, the promotion of comfort becomes the primary goal of medical management. Palliative-care teams and consultants who focus on providing symptom management to decrease suffering at the end of life have become commonplace in major teaching hospitals. The effective treatment of pain and other symptoms such as nausea, vomiting, diarrhea, and constipation play an important role in alleviating suffering in a dying child. Palliative-care clinicians also devote considerable effort to helping the child and family cope with the process of dying. At the present time, pediatric palliative-care specialists are not available for the care of all terminally ill children; therefore, many clinicians need to acquire the knowledge and skills to be able to provide these important services to gravely ill children and their families.

Children need to be helped to identify those things that matter most to them during this period. Some children wish to be with friends, read books, draw pictures, write memoirs, play with dolls or stuffed animals, or visit Disneyland. It takes time and sensitivity to help children articulate these desires; it is critical that the clinical team and family work together to do so.

Families must also determine where their terminally ill child will spend their last days of life. Many children and their families will experience a less traumatic and more comfortable death at home than in the hospital. Home hospice services can be very helpful to facilitate the transition home. Taking the child home can decrease the family's feelings of helplessness, and increase their sense of independence and responsibility. Families need help to learn about how to manage symptoms at home, including the signs and symptoms associated with impending death. Clinicians need to have a discussion about what the family should do when the child appears to be actually dying. The family needs the phone numbers of nurses or doctors available 24 hours per day who can help them with questions and support them at the actual end of the child's life; and they will need to know how the child will be declared dead at home. Also, families should have an out-of-hospital do-not-resuscitate order so that everyone involved will know that they should not intervene to prolong the dying process. Families need to be counseled not to call emergency services or an ambulance as the child is dying because emergency medical personnel may respond and intubate the dying child (regardless of the do-not-resuscitate order) and transport him or her to the hospital.

If the dying child cannot go home or if the family is unable to cope with a terminally ill child at home, the hospital and healthcare professionals should create a private and supportive environment in the medical setting that allows the family maximal contact with the child and involvement with the process of dying. Death in the midst of loved ones and without the burdens of technological intervention is certainly possible in a hospital setting.

SUPPORTING THE FAMILY AFTER THE DEATH OF A CHILD

Pediatricians can play an important role in counseling and supporting families after the death of a child. Although every death is painful to those loving family members left to grieve, perhaps the most painful death is the death of a child. The death of a child has a unique and devastating effect on the family. Even when the family has participated in a long and complicated illness and has tried to prepare for the death, grief can be profound and overwhelming.

Parents usually respond initially with a deep sense of guilt and anger. They may blame themselves, the doctors and nurses, and God for abandoning their child and allowing him or her to die. Parents also feel the acute separation from the hospital and its caregivers after the death of their child. As painful as the illness has been, the regular visits to the hospital; the talks with doctors, nurses, and social workers; and reflecting about the ups and downs of the treatment with other family members and friends has provided structure and purpose to their lives for a significant period of time. All these rituals and relationships become abruptly altered when the child's death finally occurs. Parents may feel isolated and alone with their grief. Friends may not know how to console parents who have lost a child, so they choose to distance themselves and not interact; they may provide inappropriate counsel with comments like, "at least he isn't suffering anymore," or "the baby is in a better place," or "you will get over it."

What can pediatric professionals do to help the grief stricken parents and the siblings of a child who has died? Around the time of death, mementos can be gathered to make sure that no personal items like stuffed animals, get well cards, and drawings are lost. With parental permission, pictures can be taken of the child free of attached monitors and machines. A lock of hair, and footprints and handprints from infants can be obtained. Initially after the death, the most important thing clinicians can do is to be present, to listen, to answer any questions, to say that we are sorry for their loss, and to promise to be available during the long course of grieving. Families may need to be put in touch with clergy, helped with funeral arrangements, and provided with names of community agencies that can help with costs. Most children's hospitals have pediatric bereavement programs that are available to provide counseling resources, names of community self-help support organizations, and referral services.

Pediatricians can help with counseling about what to say to siblings about the death, how siblings should be involved in the wake and funeral, and what the parents may expect as siblings express their own sadness and cope with the profound sadness of their parents. Siblings will often feel guilt at having survived or having had negative thoughts about the child who has died. Young children usually associate death with the elderly, and when a sibling dies they are often confused and frightened, fearing that they or their parents might be just as vulnerable. Some families misinterpret a sibling's lack of expressed concern about the death of their brother or sister for disinterest.

Parents often seek to protect siblings by keeping them apart from the rituals of mourning, but children are often better off being involved in funeral activities and encouraged to express their feelings. Some siblings remember, years later, the pain of feeling excluded from funeral services. If a child has never been to a funeral or burial, their fantasies about what happens may be much more upsetting than being allowed to attend. If they do attend, a close relative or friend of the family might be asked to be with the child to answer questions and to help him or her deal with their feelings.

There is no way to judge how long the acute phase of the grieving process will last for parents. Many religions acknowledge a year of grieving for a lost loved one, but when a child has died the duration of profound grief may be much longer. The anniversary of the death as well as holidays and family events like births, weddings, graduations, and even vacations, can reawaken and intensify the grief. Pediatricians can be involved in assessing the parents and siblings for pathologic or complicated grief—a condition in which grief is so profound and prolonged that serious depression, thoughts of suicide, or inability to perform the normal activities of everyday living such as keeping the house clean, cooking, working, or going to school occurs. In those circumstances, referral for mental health evaluation and treatment is needed.

Parents of children who have died are a good source of information and advice about how to provide better services and care in children's hospitals and pediatric services. Some may even be capable of counseling other families. The death of a child is always a profound and tragic loss; it is the responsibility of the healthcare community to provide the needed support and counseling to help families deal with this heartbreaking experience and continue on with their lives.

ADDITIONAL READINGS

American Academy of Pediatrics Clinical Report. Guidelines for the determination of brain death in infants and children. *Pediatrics*, 2011;128: e720–4740.

American Academy of Pediatrics Committee on Bioethics. Ethical controversies in organ donation after circulatory death. *Pediatrics*, 2013; 131:1021–1026.

American Academy of Pediatrics Committee on Hospital Care and Institute for Patient- and Family-Centered Care. Patient- and family-centered care and the pediatrician's role. *Pediatrics*, 2012; 129: 394–404.

Council on Ethical and Judicial Affairs, American Medical Association. Decisions near the end of life. *JAMA*, 1992; 267: 2229–2233.

Fleischman AR, Nolan K, Dubler NN, Epstein MF, et al. Caring for gravely ill children. *Pediatrics*, 1994; 94: 433–439.

Nelson LJ, Rushton CH, Cranford RE, Nelson RM, et al. Foregoing medically provided nutrition and hydration in pediatric patients. *J Law, Med, Ethics*, 1995; 23: 33–46.

Solomon MZ, Sellers DE, Heller KS, Dokken D, et al. New and lingering controversies in pediatric end-of-life care. *Pediatrics*, 2005; 116: 872–883.

Steele RG, Nelson TD, Cole BP. Psychosocial functioning of children with AIDS and HIV infection: review of the literature from a socioecological framework. *J Dev Behav Pediatrics*, 2007; 28: 58–69.

Truog RD, Miller FG. Changing the conversation about brain death. *Am J Bioethics*, 2014; 14: 9–14.

Wender E, and American Academy of Pediatrics Committee on Psychosocial Aspects of Child and Family Health. Supporting the family after the death of a child. Pediatrics, 2012; 130: 1164–1169.

CHAPTER 7

Ethical Issues in General Pediatric Practice

Case 1

Priscilla Cramden is a 1-year-old girl whose family recently moved to town. Her parents sought care for her with Dr. Patricia Spector, a young pediatrician in a large pediatric group practice. Although Priscilla has seen another pediatrician regularly prior to moving to this community, her parents have continually refused to allow Priscilla to be immunized. They have come to this conclusion based on fear that immunizations may cause learning disorders and autism in otherwise healthy children. They maintain that the risks of these neurodevelopmental problems are far greater for Priscilla than the risk of acquiring any of the diseases for which there are effective vaccines.

Case 2

Mrs. Carol Cruz and her daughter, Maria, came to see Dr. Patricia Spector for an annual checkup. Although there are no problems with Maria, Mrs. Cruz is anxious to talk to Dr. Spector about Jane Bartholomew, a 5-year-old girl whose family lives three houses down the block from the Cruz home. Mrs. Cruz reports that she learned from Mrs. Bartholomew that Jane is very ill, has been running a high fever for several days, has a very swollen belly, and is vomiting everything that she is taking in. Mrs. Cruz is concerned because Jane's parents are Christian Scientists and refuse to take Jane to see a doctor. Mrs. Cruz is very worried about Jane and wonders what Dr. Spector can do to help.

Mrs. Sara Schwartz, the mother of a 15-year-old boy, Misha, calls his pediatrician, Dr. Patricia Spector, to discuss Misha's upcoming office visit. Mrs. Schwartz wants Dr. Spector to do a urine drug screen on Misha without informing him. She explains that Misha's school performance has dropped off, he has become quite surly, and he is running around with the "wrong" kind of kids who she thinks smoke pot and take drugs. She has spoken with Misha about his behavior, but he doesn't respond to her. She believes if the doctor can confirm her suspicions about drug use, she can be more affective in limiting Misha's social interactions and assuring that he stops abusing drugs. She fears that if Misha is told about the drug testing, he will refuse the test, be furious with her, and act out even more negatively.

Ethical dilemmas are not only found in pondering issues at the beginning and end of life in neonatal and pediatric intensive care units or on the oncology ward. Primary-care physicians in the everyday practice of pediatrics frequently face difficult situations in which value conflicts or perceived conflicts in duties and obligations arise that affect the interests of patients and families. These situations can be divided into two groups: those that directly relate to an individual physician's relationship to patients and families, and those that place the physician in conflict because of relationships with others such as employers, insurers, or industry. In either case, pediatricians must confront their own values and beliefs about what is the right course of action. This analysis is based on the perception that physicians are moral agents, responsible for their actions, not just in the medical and scientific areas, but also in the ethical sphere.

Physician integrity, the ability to incorporate strongly held personal values into professional conduct, is fundamental to the practice of medicine. Medical practice should embody a set of scientific and humanistic principles, the goals of which are to benefit patients. A pediatrician's personal views of a particular patient's best interest are important and should be respected, even when they conflict with the views of others concerned with the patient's well-being. First we will explore some common conflicts that practicing pediatricians face in relationships with patients and families: parental refusal of medically indicated immunizations and treatments, reporting of suspected child abuse and neglect to state child-protection agencies, requests by patients and families for tests and treatments that are not medically indicated, and physician conscientious-based objections to provide medical treatments that are legally available but personally objectionable. We will then discuss value conflicts inherent in pediatricians' relationships with employers, insurers and industry.

PARENTAL REFUSAL OF ROUTINE IMMUNIZATIONS

Routine immunization of infants and young children is one of the most important public health successes of the 20th century, resulting in the estimated prevention of over 3 million deaths per year worldwide. Immunization against smallpox is no longer needed because the virus and its devastating disease have been completely eradicated. Polio epidemics raged each summer in the United States in the mid-20th century and resulted in death and disability for thousands of children. Through vaccination, the disease is now exceedingly rare. Haemophilus influenza vaccine has dramatically reduced the incidence of often-fatal cases of bacterial meningitis and epiglottitus. Immunization against diphtheria, tetanus, measles, mumps, and rubella, has made these illnesses so rare as to be virtually unrecognizable by young clinicians. Pertussis immunization resulted in the near elimination of that disease until recent childhood outbreaks and even deaths due to the transmission of Pertussis to young infants by adult caregivers whose susceptibility to infection increased because of waning antibody protection. The current recommended immunization regimen requires over 20 injections during the first year of life, and more as the child grows older, in order to prevent over a dozen very serious childhood diseases. Overall, U.S. vaccination rates exceed 90% for most recommended vaccines among children entering kindergarten. Yet, there is substantial geographic variation with parents in some communities refusing to vaccinate their children, and increasing hesitancy among parents generally, to allow some or all vaccinations to be administered to their children.

It is not surprising that the successful elimination of so many serious diseases in our communities has resulted in complacency among many parents and some physicians about the critical importance of routine vaccinations. Surveys note that 70% of pediatricians have at least one parent refuse immunization of their child each year, with some regions of the country having much higher rates of refusal. Remarkably, 4% of pediatricians admitted to having refused an immunization for their own child. The combination measles-mumps-rubella (MMR) vaccine is refused most frequently, with refusal of varicella (chickenpox) immunization the next most common. Why are parents refusing recommended immunizations and what should clinicians do about this problem?

Most parents are concerned that their young children will experience the discomfort of receiving many painful injections. Some parents have strongly held religious convictions that preclude any medications being administered to their family members. Others just don't trust information provided by the medical profession. But most parents refuse immunizations for their children because they believe the benefits of immunization do not outweigh what they believe to be the considerable risks. In any risk-benefit analysis, one must weigh the potential benefits of a treatment against the known risks of that treatment, as well as the risks of not receiving the treatment.

The benefits of immunization programs are substantial. Before children were routinely immunized in the United States, each year 15,000 died of diphtheria, 12,000 suffered from meningitis, and 8,000 suffered from pneumonia due to Haemophilus. Thousands were hospitalized and some died from polio, pertussis, and measles. But today, with most children immunized, even an unimmunized child has much less risk of becoming infected with these diseases. Because of "herd immunity" due to routine immunization programs, the infectious agents are less prevalent in the community and there is less likelihood of a susceptible child being exposed to one of these disease causing viruses and bacteria. The unimmunized child becomes a "free-rider," benefitting from whatever risks are encountered by those around him who do comply with recommended immunizations. Thus, some families are willing to place personal interests and concerns ahead of civil responsibility; they disregard their duty to participate in public-health programs that have a generally accepted level of individual risk but benefit all members of the community.

What are the current risks of not being immunized and what are the known risks of the currently used vaccines? The current risk of being unimmunized depends on the environment in which the child lives, plays, and travels; it depends on the probability of contracting a preventable illness and the morbidity and mortality associated with that infection. Unimmunized children at greatest risk for disease are those who live in communities with many other unimmunized children. Outbreaks of measles in private schools and camps populated by children from religious communities who shun immunization have resulted in a significant incidence of disease in those children and even some deaths. CDC data reveals serious increases in morbidity and mortality for unimmunized infants hospitalized with pertussis, haemophilus meningitis, and meningococcemia.

A recent review of vaccine safety examined a 2011 Institute of Medicine report and additional relevant studies, as well as practice statements, package inserts, and manufacturer information packets from vaccines. Careful examination of safety data related to MMR vaccine confirmed prior reports that the strength of evidence is high that receipt of MMR vaccine is not associated with the onset of autism or leukemia in children. Data do reveal that fever post MMR immunization sporadically is associated with benign febrile seizures in otherwise normal children, and that there is an increased incidence of these and other adverse events in immunodeficient children who receive the vaccines. Adverse events after other routine immunizations are very unusual and clinically mild except for the problem of intussusception found rarely after administration of vaccines to prevent rotavirus. These reports conclude that the protective benefits of recommended vaccination programs in the normal population far outweighs the risk of any adverse event.

Priscilla, the unimmunized 1-year-old in Case 1, who presented to Dr. Spector for well-child care, was found to be a healthy thriving child. But, Priscilla's parents refused routine immunizations when offered, based on their view that such treatments are unnecessary, could be harmful, and therefore, not in Priscilla's best interest. Dr. Spector felt that they had two false assumptions that required discussion. First, Dr. Spector shared the data that the risk of serious illness is substantial in an unimmunized child. She described the risk of meningitis and pertussis in infants, and the recent epidemics of measles among preschool children. She also attempted to reassure the parents that there are no data to support an association between immunization and autism or other serious diseases, and that the chance of adverse events postvaccination is very low. Although the Cramdens listened politely, and told Dr. Spector that they liked and respected her, they did not change their mind about immunizing Priscilla. Dr. Spector was concerned about her patient's well-being and discussed this problem with the other physicians in her group. Two senior pediatricians recommended that after another try to convince the parents to allow immunization, Dr. Spector should "fire" the patient, refusing to care for her, and suggesting that the family seek care elsewhere. They based this recommendation on three concerns: first, if the family could not trust the doctor's view concerning immunization, it was likely they would show poor compliance with other recommended medical tests and treatments in the future; second, having an unimmunized child visiting the practice placed other patients in the waiting room at increased risk for contracting illnesses such as pertussis, haemophilus, and measles for which they were not yet fully immunized; and, third, the practice might risk liability if Priscilla or other patients became ill with vaccine-preventable diseases.

My recommendation to primary-care physicians in this situation is different from the recommendation made by the senior partners in Dr. Spector's practice. I believe that, first, clinicians should listen carefully to parents who are refusing to accept routine immunizations and explore in a nonjudgmental manner their motivation for this decision. We need to ensure that cost is not a motivation for refusal. The cost of completely immunizing an infant is considerable. Parents often believe that pediatricians are making a great deal of money on these shots. We need to explain to parents that the cost of vaccination is high due to the price of the drugs themselves, not due to the price of the administration of the shots. Although private insurance coverage and Medicaid are supposed to reimburse for vaccinations, clinicians should review family insurance plans to assure that parents are not unduly burdened by any additional expenses. If needed, arrangements should be made for the child to be immunized at a local free public health clinic. If parents complain about the numbers of shots per visit or the frequency of shots, clinicians can agree to somewhat alter or extend the immunization timetable to accommodate these concerns, although this practice is not recommended.

Next, parents need to be informed about local laws concerning child care, preschool, and kindergarten requirements for immunization before admission. Exemption rules and processes vary widely. Parents may wish to consider the problems and consequences of being unable to find child care or a pre-K school for their unimmunized child, and they will need to understand how difficult it will be for their child to enter school without a modicum of vaccinations. Although most states allow exemption from immunization for religious reasons, less than half allow exemption on personal philosophical grounds.

Clinicians should ask parents how they learned about the risks of immunization. I think parents should be informed about the misleading publication in *Lancet* in 1998 by Andrew Wakefield, a British physician, who began much of the concern about the risk of MMR vaccination. This article concluded that immunization with the triple MMR vaccine at 12 months was associated with the development of a pervasive developmental disorder resembling autism. The article recommended that single-dose vaccines be used. Additional papers from the same author continued to argue that routine immunization with MMR was unsafe. After these publications, rates of immunization dropped significantly in England and the United States. Subsequently, it was revealed that Wakefield's data had been manipulated or fabricated, and that serious financial conflicts of interest may have motivated him to advocate for single dose vaccines over the available triple dose MMR. The *Lancet* partially retracted the paper in 2004, and fully retracted it in 2010. The author was found guilty of professional medical misconduct and his license to practice medicine was revoked.

In the United States, a few prominent celebrities have promoted the idea that vaccination is associated with the development of autism. One such figure, Jennie McCarthy, a model, actress, and television personality, became an antivaccination activist after her son developed autism. Because of her access to the media, millions of young parents read about or heard her view that infants who are immunized risk serious developmental abnormalities. This admired public figure convinced many American parents not to immunize their children. It is important for pediatricians to dispute this misinformation by addressing the issue directly. Physicians should explain to a parent that they personally have heard the argument on TV or viewed it on YouTube and agree that the speaker appears earnest and convincing. But clinicians should go on to state unequivocally that based on all of the available scientific and epidemiologic data, the information being conveyed by people like Jennie McCarthy is factually wrong and dangerous. For some parents, distributing articles about this issue can be helpful.

Clinicians also need to be honest and admit that immunization is not completely risk free. Like all medical tests and treatments, vaccinations are associated with some risks, but these risks are rare, and not nearly as severe as the risks of the diseases we aim to prevent. We need to remind parents that the reason they have not seen the ravages of these diseases is precisely because of universal immunization programs, and that they should ask their parents or grandparents to recall polio or measles epidemics they experienced decades ago, or to remember the child who died of meningitis in their community. Additionally, the doctor may wish to tell the story of an infant who died recently in their community or a nearby one from pertussis or meningitis, reminding parents that although these diseases are preventable, there are few treatments that can affect the course of illness once the child has become infected. This may be a compelling way to shake the firmness of parental convictions. This approach allows parents to know that the physician has evaluated the information carefully, that the medical and scientific community have taken it seriously, and have overwhelmingly agreed on the benefits and relative safety of immunization. It is hoped that this approach will encourage an open dialogue and enhance trust and respect between the doctor and parents.

If parents continue to refuse vaccination, documentation in the medical record of the reasons and of the extent of discussion is important. Repeatedly addressing this issue is also important, but it should be done in a way that does not alienate the family and decrease the likelihood that they will continue to bring the child in for care. I do not believe that pediatric practices should sever their relationships with families that continue to refuse vaccination. "Firing" the family is counterproductive since it rarely results in the child being vaccinated, it is unlikely to decrease liability risks (that are low to begin with), it eliminates the opportunity for continued respectful dialogue about this issue, and there are other ways to protect vulnerable young infants from exposure to unvaccinated patients in the office.

PARENTAL REFUSAL OF MEDICALLY INDICATED TREATMENTS ON RELIGIOUS GROUNDS

Parents or guardians are generally the appropriate decision-makers for treatment decisions for their children. Parents are charged with the responsibility of determining what best promotes the child's interests and should be given broad latitude to integrate cultural, religious, and personal values into these assessments. However, parents, in making surrogate decisions for their children, are not given the same deference or level of autonomous choice as adults who make decisions for themselves. Parents should not be permitted to refuse clearly beneficial medical treatments such as antibiotics for bacterial meningitis or surgery for bowel obstruction, without which the child is likely to suffer serious and irrevocable harm or even death.

The vast majority of Americans believe that religion plays an important role in their lives and that their children should be exposed to religious education and practice. What are the limits of respect for religious beliefs and practices when they come in conflict with the provision of medically indicated treatments for children?

There are about 100,000 individuals in the United States who identify themselves as believers in Christian Science, a religious sect that teaches that it is God's will for people to be healthy, to not suffer, to be sick, or to die. They believe that God is all- powerful and ever present, and that prayer can be as effective as medical treatments to heal those who are sick. There are other, smaller, groups in the United States whose members refuse medical care for themselves and their children. Additionally, there are some individuals who hold personal moral beliefs that preclude the use of physicians and medicines.

Physicians who care for children are given the responsibility to make independent assessments of the best interest of their patients, and to advocate for their patient when parents refuse known efficacious treatments. However, children in families who practice Christian Science do not present to healthcare providers for care. Jane Bartholomew, the five-year-old girl in Case 2 in this chapter, likely has never seen a physician or received an immunization. Dr. Spector has no professional relationship to Jane or her parents, and may wish to ignore what is likely to be a very difficult situation. But as a knowledgeable physician and concerned community member, Dr. Spector should get involved. Dr. Spector could encourage Jane's neighbor, Mrs. Cruz, to anonymously contact the state child protective services agency and should give her the hotline number to call. Suspicion of a problem, reported by a neighbor, should be investigated by the agency. If Mrs. Cruz is reluctant to make the call, since Dr. Spector has now learned that Jane may be suffering from a treatable illness that, if untreated, could result in death or serious disability, Dr. Spector should place the call based solely on the information she has heard from Mrs. Cruz. Although we should respect the right of families to hold any or no religious beliefs, our society does not allow parents to harm their children based on these religious beliefs. Since the mid-20th century, courts have consistently ruled that the right to practice religion freely does not extend to exposing children to ill health or death. Although adults may martyr themselves based on religious beliefs, they may not make martyrs of their children.

Each state has laws setting out the obligations of healthcare professionals to report suspected child abuse or neglect. When a physician or nurse suspects that a child is seriously ill and may suffer irrevocable harm, and the family is not seeking medical care for that child, there is a legal and moral obligation to report this situation to the state child-protective-services agency. Such agencies have the responsibility to urgently investigate suspected abuse and neglect and, if needed, to bring the child to medical attention. Most state medical-neglect statutes would empower the authorities to remove the sick child from the home and bring him or her to the hospital for care. Generally, the parents would not be held criminally negligent for refusing to seek care for their child due to a "religious exemption" in the law for those whose religious beliefs preclude interaction with the medical establishment. The American Academy of Pediatrics and other child advocates have recommended that religious exemptions in child-abuse and neglect laws be repealed so that all children are equally protected. I share that view. Additionally, this change would reduce confusion about the duty to report abuse and neglect and to obtain treatment for sick children. Healthcare professionals should report suspected cases of medical neglect to state child-protection agencies regardless of whether or not the parents' decision is based on religious beliefs.

REPORTING SUSPECTED CHILD ABUSE AND NEGLECT

A more common problem in general pediatric practice is the observation that a patient may have been abused or is being neglected. Close to a million children and adolescents in the United States are confirmed each year to have suffered from neglect, or physical, sexual, and emotional abuse. Allowing for failures of detection and underreporting, the actual incidence of these problems is far greater. Child abuse and neglect affect children of all ages, ethnicities, religions, and socioeconomic groups. The consequences of abuse and neglect are serious and long standing, including severe illness and disability as well as death. In addition, mental illness and social and behavioral disorders are a common consequence of abuse, and those who have suffered from abuse are more likely to perpetrate abuse in the future. Why are pediatricians and other health professionals failing to detect these serious problems in children, and when detected, why are they reluctant to report these cases to state authorities?

Child abuse and neglect most often occurs in dysfunctional families who struggle with mental illness, domestic violence, illicit drug use, poverty, and overcrowding. A child who presents to a healthcare professional with signs of injury or failure to reach expected weight or growth parameters should raise concerns about possible abuse or neglect. Although these problems can be associated with many possible causes, abuse and neglect should be in the differential diagnosis. It is often difficult to assess whether an injury is accidental or inflicted. It is helpful to take a careful history of the events that led to the injury, to consider if the explanation of the cause is consistent with the nature of the injury, whether the explanation changes over time, and whether the explanation is possible based on the child's age and developmental abilities. The child and other witnesses may also be helpful in confirming what occurred.

A general medical history including past injuries, compliance with preventive health and immunization visits, and family history of bone and bleeding disorders is important. In addition, knowledge of recent emotional, social, and financial stressors in the family can be helpful. The physical examination is important. The child should be completely undressed and carefully examined. Cuts, bruises, bites, and other skin injuries can suggest abuse. Examination of all bones, including ribs and extremities may reveal new, healing or old fractures. Serious dental caries, diaper rash, and overall poor hygiene may point to a child who has been neglected. Examination of the external areas around the anus and genitalia can reveal signs of sexual abuse. All findings need to be documented accurately. The general pediatrician may need x-rays, laboratory tests, and consultation from experts in child abuse, orthopedics, neurology, hematology, and other specialties in order to validate suspicions of abuse.

A report of suspected child abuse or neglect is not based on certainty of the diagnosis, but rather on suspicion. Healthcare professionals are legally obligated to report suspected child abuse and neglect. However, they are frequently reluctant to report suspected maltreatment for fear of insulting the family, potentially losing the patient, and most importantly, of being wrong and inflicting the trauma of an unnecessary investigation on the family. Every family found to have a reasonable suspicion of child abuse and neglect is subjected to a thorough investigation by state child protection agency staff. This process can be quite onerous and may generate significant anxiety and concern within the family. During the investigation, the child might remain at home or with relatives or he or she might be placed in temporary foster care. The goal of the investigation is to provide evidence of abuse or neglect in order to obtain needed services and treatments for the child, and to assess what services might be provided to the family in order to prevent further abuse. Sometimes the result of the investigation is the conclusion that the child should not remain with the family on a temporary or permanent basis.

Perhaps another even more troubling reason for hesitancy in reporting suspected cases of abuse is the concern that the child-protection agencies do less than an optimal job of assessing families and providing services and interventions that are helpful to children and families. Agencies frequently lack adequately trained staff and sufficient resources to provide services to help families mitigate the problems that have caused the abuse or neglect in the first place. It is also feared that placing a child in foster care may not be a positive experience that enhances the child's future. Although the vast majority of foster-care families are caring and supportive, some children report negative and even abusive experiences in foster care.

The child-protection system is imperfect, but I believe pediatricians should fulfill their legal, moral, and professional obligations to report suspected child abuse and neglect, and then work closely with the agencies responsible for investigating the allegations. Healthcare professionals should explain to families that the law requires reporting when children are injured and the circumstances are unclear. It is important that the state protect our children by reviewing each situation when circumstances suggest a child may be in danger. Pediatricians need to play a significant role in advocating for the services needed by dysfunctional families and stressed parents; and healthcare professionals need to work with foster care agencies to help families reunite when possible.

PHYSICIAN REFUSAL TO PROVIDE REQUESTED TESTS OR TREATMENTS

Healthcare professionals sometimes refuse to provide tests or treatments that they believe are not appropriate based on medical indications, patient interests, or their personal conscience. Physicians are moral agents, responsible for their own behaviors. They should act in ways that they believe to be in their patient's interests and not antithetical to their own professional and personal values. When may a physician refuse to provide a medical test or treatment?

Physicians are often asked by parents to provide antibiotics, in addition to symptomatic treatment, for children with viral illnesses who will not benefit from antibiotic treatment. Parents may be motivated by the belief that antibiotics will make their child feel better and will be effective in shortening the length of illness. They may also be concerned that if the child does not improve with symptomatic treatment and the viral illness evolves into a bacterial one, they will be faced with the inconvenience and cost associated with a return visit to the physician's office. Physicians should resist the easy way out and should not comply with a parent's request for medication that is not indicated. From a medical perspective, administering antibiotics when not indicated increases the risk of known side effects such as rash, gastrointestinal disturbances, and acute allergic reactions. Inappropriate use of antibiotics also increases the likelihood of the development of antibiotic resistance among bacteria, heightening the threat of serious illness in the broader community. This type of refusal to provide a requested treatment requires the physician to spend time and effort to educate the parents, and to explain why it is inappropriate to comply with their request. Although this may be time consuming, it is the ethically and professionally appropriate approach to this problem. Physicians who comply with these requests are placing their patients and their communities at undue risk, and are acting in a manner that is inconsistent with good and accepted medical practice.

A more complicated issue arises when a parent requests that the physician surreptitiously obtain a urine sample from their child to test for drugs of abuse. Misha, the 15-year-old in Case 3 in this chapter, has exhibited decreased school performance and surly behavior, and he has been associating with adolescents whom his mother believes are taking illicit drugs. She asks her pediatrician to surreptitiously test her son's urine for drugs of abuse in an effort to use these data to confront Misha and help change his behavior. She fears that if the doctor asks Misha's permission to do the testing, he will refuse, get angry at his mother, and intensify his acting-out behaviors. What should Dr. Spector, the pediatrician, do?

The recreational use of illicit and prescription drugs among adolescents is increasing. Marijuana for medical and recreational use is becoming legalized in states throughout the country. Adolescents have always experimented with alcohol and drugs and have suffered significant morbidity and mortality from these practices. Pediatricians play a significant role in partnering with parents and schools to deter, detect, and treat drug and alcohol abuse in children. Dr. Spector, Misha's pediatrician, knew that covert drug testing is a poor substitute for developing open communication and voluntary cooperation from her patient in order to understand what is going on in his life. Drug testing is an adjunct to a thorough history, not a replacement. Drug testing also has limits. Although urine samples may reveal drugs of abuse taken several days or even weeks prior to the test, a negative result does not rule out drug use. Since some drugs are eliminated from the body fairly quickly, if illicit use occurs on weekends, a sample of urine provided on the following Thursday or Friday may test negative. Also, since adolescents are aware that urine may be tested for illicit substances, when asked to provide a sample, they may substitute another person's urine, or dilute their own urine, or add chemicals to the sample to make testing inaccurate. There are also false positive results from urine screening. Some prescribed medications and even some foods may cross react with illicit drug metabolites to result in a positive test.

I believe healthcare professionals should sympathize with parents' concerns about illicit drug use, but should not agree to surreptitious urine testing. Rather, the pediatrician should strive to develop a relationship with the adolescent that will allow an open dialogue about these issues. If the adolescent denies using drugs, then voluntary urine testing can be suggested to help calm parents' concerns. If the child admits to using drugs, testing can be suggested to help sort out what he is actually taking since street drugs often contain chemicals other than those suspected. If the pediatrician has obtained a thorough history and believes she has sufficient information to initiate treatment or referral, testing may not be indicated.

It is also important for the pediatrician to discuss with her patient what she will tell his parents about their communication. Adolescents need to be viewed as partners in their care. Confidentiality should be maintained if the adolescent is not behaving in ways that directly jeopardize their health and well-being. But confidentiality may be breached and parents and others may need to be involved in care when serious problems like illicit drug use exist. Openness and honesty with the adolescent patient is important in order to maintain trust and to enhance the therapeutic relationship that is needed for an optimal outcome.

In addition to refusing to provide a test or treatment because it is not medically indicated or not in the patient's interest, physicians sometimes refuse to provide a medical treatment based on a conscience-based objection. A conscience-based objection results from strongly held moral, religious, or political beliefs. Physicians may wish to invoke conscience-based objections in order to refuse to: provide a particular treatment, treat a particular person, inform a patient about certain legally available treatments, or refer a patient to other physicians who might agree to provide such treatments. When pediatricians invoke claims of conscience, it is generally related to refusing to provide treatment or referral in the areas of abortion, sterilization, and contraception. These are highly charged issues that often relate to strongly held religious or philosophical beliefs concerning abstinence, the moral status of an embryo or fetus, and the primary role of reproduction in marriage. Since pediatric patients are children and adolescents, the strength of conscientious objection to refuse participation in these areas of medical treatment may be even greater than when dealing with adults.

There are morally important reasons to protect a physician's right to exercise conscience-based objections to treatment, even if we disagree with the content or basis of the refusal. Performing an action that violates a person's conscience undermines his or her sense of integrity and self-respect. It is important to the practice of medicine that physicians maintain their integrity and self-respect as they interact with patients and colleagues. But the core ethical principles and professional obligations of medicine justify some constraints on conscience objections. Clinicians have beneficence-based obligations to promote the health and well-being of their patients. We are obligated to maximize benefits and minimize harms for patients while we respect their autonomous choices. These obligations constrain conscience objections.

I believe society and healthcare institutions should respect the right of a physician to invoke conscience-based objections that relate to recommending, performing, or prescribing abortion, sterilization, or contraceptive services, but that physicians must fulfill their duty to inform patients about available options and alternatives, or to refer patients for such information, so the patient's rights and well-being are not harmed. If a physician is unwilling to fulfill his duty to inform or refer, he should not be allowed to continue to see patients who might need these services. In addition, I believe that physicians are obligated to inform their patients and their employers of any strongly held beliefs or practices that may affect the care of some patients in their practice. Physicians and the institutions in which they work should be held accountable to ensure that respect for conscience objections does not negatively affect patients.

PHYSICIANS AS EMPLOYEES

More than two-thirds of the physicians who care for children are employed by hospitals, health systems, clinics, or large group practices. The era of the solo practitioner depicted in the classic Norman Rockwell paintings of the mid-20th century is no longer an accurate representation of the general practice of pediatrics. Increasing costs of office administration and malpractice insurance and decreasing reimbursement from insurers, as well as contemporary business strategies of hospitals and health systems, have resulted in most pediatricians becoming salaried physicians in the employ of larger corporate entities. Becoming an employee can liberate physicians from the obligations of running a business and allow them to focus on their chosen profession. But there are potential problems that can occur when physicians are faced with obligations to their patients that may be in conflict with the interests of their employer. This problem of "dual agency" can result in serious ethical concerns.

Physicians like to take responsibility, trust their knowledge and intuition, and tend to enjoy functioning independently. The work of being a doctor is central to their identity and provides continual opportunities to do good. Medicine is a profession and physicians are professionals. As such, physicians have a fiduciary relationship to each patient, and patients may expect and trust that a physician in good faith has a duty to act solely in their interests. The profession of medicine is given a quasi monopoly to practice medicine by the state with the expectation that each physician will be adequately educated, will provide competent care, and will behave in an ethical manner. The state allows the profession to determine its own educational curriculum, certifying examinations, and ethical standards, and to be responsible for holding its practitioners accountable through professional boards of conduct.

But when physicians become employees, they also have a clear duty of loyalty to their employers. Employment, in and of itself, does not threaten the spirit or ethos of professionalism. The American Medical Association Code of Ethics recognizes the potential for conflict in dual agency and explicitly states that a physician's paramount responsibility is to his or her patient, even when a physician has a duty of loyalty to an employer. Patient interests and welfare must take priority, and treatment and referral decisions should always be based on the best interest of the patient. How should physicians act when employers create rules that limit the use of certain expensive drugs, devices, or tests, or limit referrals for imaging or specialty care to physicians also employed by the institution? Will physicians jeopardize their future employment if they break the rules?

Employers have a right to expect that their employees will be loyal and abide by the rules of their organization. Hospitals have always employed professionals such as lawyers, but a lawyer employed by a hospital has a fiduciary responsibility to the hospital as her client, whereas a physician employed by the hospital has hundreds of patients as her clients and does not have a fiduciary responsibility to the hospital. Hospitals, health systems, and group practices need clear and explicit policies that recognize the primary role of patient interests and allow for physician discretion in deciding on appropriate tests, drugs, treatments, and referrals. Physician-run committees to determine institutional policies that affect the quality of care and physician competence can best accomplish this. Physicians seeking employment should examine institutional policies to be certain that they are consistent with prioritizing patient interests. Physicians are at risk of being fired if they break hospital rules, even when those rules appear inappropriate and not in the interest of an individual patient. I often counsel young physicians to raise these patient- related concerns with hospital peers, appropriate committees, and chief medical officers as a way to advocate for an individual patient and, at the same time, attempt to change the rules. This approach is less likely to result in termination of employment and more likely to result in institutional change.

There is a great deal of evidence that the transformation of the average physician from a small business man with a private office to an employee of a large corporate structure is good for patients. This is a result of enhancing the general quality of care and the accountability of individual physicians. What went on in private offices was rarely open to scrutiny; what occurs in hospitals and large group practices is extensively monitored and evaluated. This results in far more evidence-based practice and better outcomes for patients.

Another beneficial change in healthcare delivery is the redefinition of who is the hospital's "customer." Thirty years ago, the private physicians who admitted their patients to hospitals were viewed as the customers of the institution; their needs and desires needed to be recognized and prioritized. Today, patients are identified as the hospital's customers, resulting in patient- and family-centered care initiatives and a focus on patient satisfaction that drive hospital policies and practices. I believe this transformation has been extraordinarily good for patients.

Clinicians in general practice are constantly reminded that their patients' source of payment is a critical part of decision making around care. Pediatricians are faced with navigating the coverage, approval systems, and practices for each of five or six major insurers in their region, and with interpreting for patients and their families the specific limits and coverage offered by their personal policy. In addition to mastering the private insurance system, pediatricians that accept Medicaid, the public insurer, must be familiar with additional rules and forms. The amount of time, personnel, and overhead costs needed to interact with this complicated reimbursement system are extraordinary. These activities take a large proportion of physician time and account for well over 50% of practice income. It is perhaps the most important reason that general pediatricians are opting to become employees, or affiliating with large group practices. The relationship of clinicians to the health-insurance system is complicated and filled with ethical concerns. How much time and effort should clinicians utilize to advocate for their patients when insurers refuse to approve indicated tests and treatments? Should clinicians game the system to obtain indicated tests and treatments for their patients? Should they outright lie for their patients? Should multiple procedures or treatments performed at a single visit be billed separately and with different dates of service in order to facilitate payment?

Patients expect that clinicians and hospitals should provide all tests and treatments that might benefit them and that their insurance should cover the costs. Physicians wish to provide all tests and treatments they believe will benefit their patients and become quite upset when insurance companies refuse to approve or pay for these indicated procedures and medications. Physicians generally see no duty of loyalty to insurers; they know that there are laws, regulations, and ethical principles that require honesty in transactions with insurers, but they often view these payers as impediments to providing the highest quality of medically indicated care to patients. Clinicians and office staff members quickly learn how to describe a patient's symptoms in the manner most likely to garner permission for a diagnostic x-ray or MRI test. Although not lying, per se, staff members learn to describe symptoms, signs, and tentative diagnoses using key words or phrases that will meet the insurer's criteria for approval and payment. Insurers can refuse to approve a requested test or treatment arguing that it is not a covered service of the policy or that the procedure is not medically indicated for the illness as described. These justifications for rejection may be questions of fact or rebuttable presumptions. Physicians should extend themselves to advocate for their patients with insurance companies. Although this has become one of the most distasteful aspects of practicing medicine, it has become more and more necessary in order to fulfill our obligations to patients.

Both clinicians and patients need to remember that, although insurers can refuse to approve or pay for a requested test, procedure, or treatment, insurers cannot preclude a physician or hospital from providing the intervention. Although expensive, patients may opt to receive an unapproved test, procedure, or treatment and pay for it themselves. However, most patients cannot afford to pay for unapproved tests or treatments, so it most often falls upon the clinician to convince insurance company staff that the requested test or treatment is medically indicated and deserves coverage. It may be acceptable to present requests for coverage in the most advantageous manner based on experience, but it is not ethical to game the system and lie for patients.

Lying for patients fundamentally harms the physician-patient relationship. This relationship is based on trust. Lying runs the risk of undermining the physician's credibility in the patient's eyes. If the doctor is willing to lie for a patient, will he or she be completely truthful to the patient under different circumstances? Lying may also exaggerate the level of illness and have unforeseen consequences for the patient concerning work-related issues and future insurance coverage. Lying may also harm others, prioritizing a less-sick patient over those who are more in need of a desired procedure, intensive-care bed or organ transplant.

Lying also breaches several fundamental duties created by the contract between physician and insurer, like the obligation to be honest, and fair. These breaches can result in significant fines and even loss of license for physicians. Although there may at first glance seem to be justifiable reasons to game the system or even lie for patients, the potential negative consequences to patient, physician, and the healthcare system argue against this practice. Physicians owe their patients competent practice, reasonable advice, and committed advocacy to fulfill their ethical and fiduciary responsibilities. Nothing more should be expected and nothing more should be offered.

RELATIONSHIPS WITH INDUSTRY

A pediatrician in general practice is likely to interact frequently with representatives of the pharmaceutical industry. Young, attractive men and women promote pharmaceutical products and infant formula directly to clinicians and staff in pediatric practices. These salespersons distribute literature for physicians and for parents, as well as pens, pads, and other branded products, and samples of new and frequently used products. Clinicians often use the pens and find it very helpful to distribute the drug samples as starter doses to distressed parents of sick children, so that they do not need to stop at the drug store on the way home. This is often greatly appreciated by parents and not seen as affecting the choice of treatment by the doctors. However, studies have shown that most clinicians receive the bulk of their education on new antibiotics from interactions with drug reps, and that prescribing practices are dramatically affected by these meetings. New, more expensive antibiotics are often prescribed for illnesses that could be effectively treated with older, less expensive drugs, despite the protestations from clinicians that they are unaffected by these interactions with sales people. The pharmaceutical industry would not be spending money on reps visiting offices if it was not economically beneficial. Pediatricians need to be wiser than to believe that their judgment and practice is not being affected by these visits. Evidence of new, effective treatments should be garnered from reputable pediatric literature and not from sales people.

The pharmaceutical industry also provides free continuing education programs for practicing physicians, inviting highly respected, well-compensated speakers to recommend or at least reference their products in the context of a lecture on the diagnosis and treatment of a common disease. These events often include cocktail receptions and elegant dinners. Such programs are expensive, but have been shown by the industry to provide excellent return on investment by positively impacting sales. Physicians are also provided with continuing medical education credits for attendance at these events, credits that are needed for license renewal in most states. National accrediting organizations and the Food and Drug Administration have created strict conflict-of-interest rules for any educational program providing continuing medical education credits that includes reference to a regulated drug or device. Yet, the pharmaceutical industry seems able to skillfully construct programs that enhance sales and fulfill the continuing education standards at least on paper. Pediatricians should avoid these programs.

A more malicious practice is the compensation of physicians for prescribing a specific drug or device to patients. An example of how this might work in a pediatric practice would be the payment of a fee to a physician who prescribes a specific drug for Attention Deficit Hyperactivity Disorder (ADHD), a commonly overdiagnosed problem that requires long-term treatment. The physician is incentivized to make the diagnosis and to prescribe a specific drug. To curtail this practice, the Physician Payments Sunshine Act was enacted by Congress in 2010 as part of the healthcare reform law. This Act is intended to provide greater transparency into the relationships between pharmaceutical and device manufacturers and healthcare providers by requiring manufacturers to report payments and other "transfers of value" provided to physicians and teaching hospitals to the Centers for Medicare and Medicaid Services (CMS). These reports are available to state boards of professional conduct and to the public through websites and other listings. Although the intention to increase transparency and shine a light on this practice is laudable, it is questionable whether it has resulted in any significant decrease in these practices. Pediatricians should not enter into the practice of being compensated by a company for prescribing a medication or device.

Physicians need to recognize that each of these types of interactions with industry create conflicts of interest, and do affect their decision-making and their fiduciary responsibilities to patients. Pediatricians in general practice must create strict personal standards for any relationships with industry representatives to ensure that their prescribing preferences and their practices are not compromised. Generally, such standards should include not accepting gifts of any kind from industry reps, not attending industry administered educational programs, and not accepting incentives to prescribe any medications.

FINAL THOUGHTS

Ethical problems are common in the general practice of pediatrics. The intimate relationships between patients, families, and their physicians, as well as the conflicts of dual agency created by the relationships between physicians and employers, insurers and industry, generate many complicated ethical concerns. General pediatricians don't often think about these as ethical dilemmas, but they need to be aware that they face these issues on a daily basis and should spend time creating thoughtful solutions to these ethical concerns.

ADDITIONAL READINGS

American Academy of Pediatrics, Committee on Bioethics. Physician refusal to provide information or treatment on the basis of claims of conscience. Pediatrics, 2009; 124: 1689–1693.

American Academy of Pediatrics Committee on Bioethics. Conflicts between religious and spiritual beliefs and pediatric care: informed refusal, exemptions, and public funding. Pediatrics, 2013; 132: 962–965.

Diekema DS. Improving childhood vaccination rates. *N Engl J Med*, 2012; 366: 391–393.

Diekema DS, and the Committee on Bioethics, American Academy of Pediatrics Clinical Report. Responding to parental refusals of immunization of children. Pediatrics, 2005; 115: 1428–1431.

Fleischman AR, Collogan L. Addressing ethical issues in everyday practice. *Pediatric Annals*, 2004; 33: 74–745.

Kellogg ND, and the Committee on Child Abuse and Neglect, American Academy of Pediatrics. Evaluation of suspected child physical abuse. *Pediatrics*, 2007; 119: 1232–1241.

Levy S, Siqueira LM, and the Committee on Substance Abuse, American Academy of Pediatrics. Testing for drugs of abuse in children and adolescents. Pediatrics, 2014; 133: e1798-e1807.

Maglione MA, Lopamudra D, Raaen L, Smith A, et al. Safety of vaccines used for routine immunization of US Children: A systematic review. *Pediatrics*, 2014; 134: 325–337.

Morreim EH. Gaming the system—dodging the rules, ruling the dodgers. Arch Intern Med, 1991; 151: 443–447.

CHAPTER 8

Ethical Issues in the Care of Adolescents

Case 1

Pamela Harrington is a 15-year-old girl whose family is of the Jehovah's Witnesses faith. She is healthy, but found to have Acute Lymphoblastic Leukemia (ALL) after a routine camp physical reveals a very elevated white blood cell count. The doctors explain to Pamela and her family that aggressive treatment of ALL is likely to result in curing the disease but the chemotherapy can cause severe anemia and thrombocytopenia that may require blood and platelet transfusions. Both Pamela and her parents want the doctors to proceed with the treatment but will refuse any blood or blood products. An independent conversation with Pamela reveals that she is a very good student, a responsible baby sitter, and quite knowledgeable about her religious faith. She enjoys proselytizing with her mother door to door in her community, and says that she fully intends to be a Jehovah's Witness as an adult.

Case 2

Gregory Lin is a 17-year-old boy who has been treated for two years for a malignant brain tumor that has not been responsive to surgical and medical treatment. Dr. Megan Charval, the oncologist caring for Gregory, has offered the family a third round of chemotherapy in an attempt to reverse the continued growth of this aggressive tumor. She is clear that she is pessimistic that the additional treatment will help. Gregory's parents, Paul and Rosalie, are anxious to proceed with the chemotherapy and do everything possible to prolong their son's life. On the other hand, Gregory does not wish to have additional treatment that will just make him sick and is not likely to reverse the course of the tumor. Gregory asks Dr. Charval for palliative care and a do-not-resuscitate order. He would like to be comfortable in his last days or weeks of life and does not want any further chemotherapy.

Adolescents are children between puberty and biologic maturity, generally 10–18 years of age. Biological, psychological, and social changes that occur from the preteen years through young adulthood, the period of adolescence, are profound and important. Everyone remembers their own adolescence as a turbulent time because there are many developmental tasks that need to be accomplished to successfully make the transition to young adulthood. Adolescents need to deal with the biological changes that occur due to hormonal surges and physical growth. They are challenged to develop a social identity, often rejecting their parents' values and significantly influenced by peers. And they need to cope with newfound sexual feelings and attempt to develop the capacity for intimacy in relationships. This is all occurring during a period that requires intense concentration on school performance, and often the initiation of work responsibilities. An important part of adolescence is the struggle to differentiate self from parents and attain independence. This process has been called individuation, a moving toward independent decision-making or evolving autonomy. Adolescents begin to take more responsibility for what they do, and who they are, and if successful, they look less to parents for validation of their choices. This transition to competence in making autonomous decisions requires practice and thoughtful parents who respect their adolescents' needs for individuation.

Adolescence is generally a time of good health, but there are many serious diseases and conditions that begin in adolescence, including malignancies, unintentional injuries, mental illness, and substance abuse. Eating disorders, including anorexia and bulimia are common, and overweight and obesity are epidemic. Adolescents often experiment with risky behaviors that can result sometimes in significant morbidity and even mortality.

Most adolescents are considered to be minors, under the legal age of majority, or the age at which individuals are presumed to be legally competent. Competence as it is used in the law is not necessarily an indication of mental ability or decisional capacity, but a legal term that enfranchises individuals and gives them the status of "adults." Competent adults are individuals who are assumed to possess a certain level of decisional capacity and are thus granted decisional and economic autonomy. Some of the rights granted to competent adults and denied to minors include the right to vote, the right to serve in the military, and the right to enter into legally binding contracts. It is possible for adults to be declared incompetent, thus losing some or all of these rights. However, adults are presumed to be competent, whereas individuals under the age of majority are presumed to be incompetent, without the need for any proof of decisional incapacity.

Some adolescents are considered "emancipated," with all of the attendant rights and responsibilities of adulthood. These emancipated minors are treated under the law as though they had reached the age of majority and are no longer under the control of parents or guardians. They may make medical decisions for themselves without any involvement of parents or guardians. Historically, minors only became emancipated when they married or enrolled in the military, and usually with some form of tacit or explicit consent on the part of their parents or guardians. However, state statutes and court rulings have also found that minors may be considered emancipated if they live apart from their parents and are financially independent or if they are pregnant or the parents of children. Children, who are runaways or throwaways, alone on the streets and fending for themselves, are not considered emancipated minors.

Through case law and statutes in many states, the "mature minor" doctrine has evolved as a means for minors with adequate decisional capacity and understanding of their medical situation to consent to treatment without parental involvement. In all states, adolescents are given the authority to consent for some medical tests, treatments, and preventive interventions because of the realization that they will not seek care if required to inform parents about their behaviors or illness. These conditions and the restrictions on treatment vary from state to state, but generally physicians are permitted to treat adolescents without parental permission for sexually transmitted diseases, pregnancy and its prevention, mental illness, and substance abuse.

The ethical justification for the emancipated minor doctrine is quite simple. If a person of any age is capable of making reasoned judgments about their own healthcare, behaving in a responsible manner, living away from their parents, and being economically independent, they should be afforded respect for autonomy consistent with being an adult. The justification of the mature minor doctrine is somewhat more complicated. Many of the adolescents who seek care for treatment of sexually transmitted diseases, substance abuse, or pregnancy have exhibited behaviors that placed them at significant health risk and about which their parents may be concerned. It might even be in the young person's interest to involve their parents in their care to ensure compliance with treatment, decrease risky behaviors, and prevent future more serious complications of illness. However, experience informs us that adolescents with these types of disorders will delay or avoid seeking medical care if they believe that their parents will be informed, even in circumstances when delay of treatment may pose a serious threat to their health. The mature-minor doctrine, when implemented by a clinician to treat a minor without parental consent, runs the risk of enraging a parent but ensures the timely and effective treatment of the young person. The clinician in these circumstances has the obligation not only to treat the teen but also to engage the adolescent in a conversation about decreasing the risky behaviors that may have resulted in the illness. Clinicians should also explore with their patient the risks and benefits of informing parents about the illness and volunteer to help the young person have that conversation.

ADOLESCENT DECISION-MAKING

How good are adolescents at making decisions concerning their own health care? Young children and adolescents develop decisional capacity as they mature. Developmental psychologists argue that children before the age of 7 learn to use words to represent objects and begin to understand causation; children from 7–12 years of age develop the capacity to appreciate multiple perspectives on an issue and can manipulate information, but they cannot understand problems in the abstract. During adolescence, children develop the ability to think abstractly and hypothetically, as would be required for choosing between options and consenting to treatment. Experimental studies have concluded that children 14 years old have the capacity to make treatment decisions for their own healthcare equivalent to adults. Adolescents who are able to weigh the risks and benefits of multiple options and manipulate hypothetical situations before making a decision as well as adults may still not possess the life experience or perspective of an older individual. Also, adolescents are more likely than adults to act impulsively, and they are more likely to be focused on their current situation, rather than future considerations. These studies do not assume that adults always make perfect or correct decisions but, rather, that older adolescents have the ability to make decisions as well as adults. Importantly, autonomous adults may refuse any medical intervention even if it is thought by the clinician not to be in the adult's best interest to forego that treatment. Adolescents who are not emancipated do not generally have the authority to refuse medical interventions that clinicians believe are clearly in their best interest.

Clinicians treating adolescents have beneficence-based obligations to their patients only to offer treatments that they believe enhance the patient's interests. These obligations also require physicians to not accept refusal of clearly beneficial treatments. This circumstance provides some level of safety to help protect mature adolescent patients faced with hard decisions about their own healthcare. Although physicians do not replace parents as the responsible decision-maker for the child, the fact that they have beneficence-based obligations to maintain their adolescent patient's interests should mediate some of the concerns about the potential for young people to behave impulsively or be less concerned with future consequences of their present decisions.

There are times, however, when physicians should accept adolescent patient's refusal of treatment. Pamela Harrington, the 15-year-old patient with Acute Lymphoblastic Leukemia in Case 1 in this chapter, refuses to accept a blood or platelet transfusion if needed during her therapy because she is a member of the Jehovah's Witnesses faith. Pamela and her family want the doctors to treat her with the most effective medical management to save her life and enhance her future well-being. However, the Jehovah's Witnesses faith, based on their interpretation of scriptures, argues for abstaining from taking blood into the body either from transfusions of whole blood or any of its major components: red blood cells, white blood cells, platelets, or plasma. The consequence to any individual who takes blood into the body includes excommunication from the faith and eternal damnation.

In general, parents are not permitted to refuse a life-sustaining treatment for their child when the treatment is highly effective and refusal will result in imminent, irreversible, and serious harm. So why is Pamela's view important? She is still a child and not emancipated. Should doctors respect Pamela's refusal to have a transfusion as they would in the case of a 25- or 65-year old person? Pamela seems to be among those adolescents with evolving autonomy that should be respected. She appears to have the capacity to weigh the risks and benefits of her actions and to make informed choices about her healthcare. Some of her treating physicians did not wish to respect Pamela's decision about transfusion, arguing that she is a child with little say in the matter, and parents may not refuse clearly beneficial life-sustaining treatment for a child. In this case, I believe that it is important to respect Pamela's values and wishes, particularly as they coincide with those of her family. Pamela's values should be respected, not in a manner identical to the values of an adult whose wishes are respected based solely on autonomy, but Pamela's wishes should be respected based on her evolving autonomy and bolstered by the agreement of her parents, her natural surrogate decision-makers. Although parents may not refuse efficacious treatments for a child who might suffer serious and irreversible damage or death as a result, in this case, because Pamela does exhibit evolving autonomy and capacity to participate in this decision, I would respect the family's refusal.

If Pamela and her family disagreed about refusing a transfusion, it would be a much more difficult case to decide. I would be reluctant to give Pamela a blood transfusion over her objection, but with her parents permission I would likely provide the needed blood in a life-threatening situation. Although Pamela is a thoughtful adolescent, the decision to allow her to die by refusing a transfusion likely to save her life, during a course of treatment with a high likelihood to cure her disease, seems inappropriate for a child— even one with evolving autonomy. Many physicians would wish to override the autonomy of an adult who might make the same decision in order to prevent an unnecessary death, but in the United States we have created a clear principle that autonomous and capacitated adults may refuse any medical intervention. This has been an important rule and it is worth respecting, but when the patient is still a child, not an autonomous and capacitated adult, we need to take other aspects of the situation into account. And conversely, if Pamela wished to be transfused, regardless of her parents' wishes, I would provide the transfusion if needed. Saving the life of a young person who wishes to live seems like the reasonable thing to do.

Conflict in decision-making for adolescents between the patient and family is rare, but certainly occurs. This most often happens in the context of an adolescent with a serious and terminal disease near the end of life, who has decided that he or she wishes to die by withholding or withdrawing treatment, whereas the family is not yet ready to forego life-sustaining treatments. Gregory Lin, the 17-year-old in Case 2 in this chapter, believes he is dying from a malignant brain tumor. He refuses any additional chemotherapy, requests palliative care and a do-not-resuscitate order, despite his parents desire to continue aggressive treatment. His doctor believes that Gregory is a mature young man, is capable of making this choice, and that the decision to forego further treatment is a reasonable option. She will counsel the family that they should respect his choice.

When accepting the decision of a patient like Gregory to stop aggressive treatment and focus on palliative interventions, it is important to be sure that the adolescent is not pathologically depressed. It is also important to have a frank and constructive conversation with the patient's parents to help understand their perspectives. I believe it is inappropriate for the parents' views about continued treatment to prevail. Most importantly, the physicians caring for Gregory should respect his choice and assist the parents to become prepared for their child's impending death. Parents should be helped to verbalize their feelings and to discuss how they envision what will happen at the time of death. They can be assured that their child will not suffer and that they can be with him until the end. Children often accept the inevitability of their death before their parents. They do not wish to prolong their dying and at the same time they wish to protect their parents from continued suffering. The goal in these cases is to bring the parents along in the process of acceptance of the death of their child so that all can agree on the course of action. A conversation with the adolescent and the parents together can be effective in finalizing decisions about withholding further treatment and how and where death will occur. Although this type of discourse is always sad and emotional, it can be very meaningful for all participants.

CONFIDENTIALITY

Most pediatric practices inform adolescent patients and their parents of the value of maintaining confidentiality between the patient and doctor, and prospectively seek parental permission to treat the child without informing the parent of intimate and private information that may be conveyed in the clinical encounter. There are many benefits of this practice but also some important limits that need to be disclosed to all parties. The obvious benefit of maintaining confidentiality by promising that private information will not be disclosed to others without authorization is the ability to obtain information of a sensitive and personal nature that may be helpful in the therapeutic relationship. In general, a person will only share sensitive and potentially damaging information with another if they can trust that person to safeguard it. In the clinical setting, such information is often critical for appropriate diagnosis and treatment of many disorders.

Although promising to maintain confidentiality with an adolescent patient, the clinician must also explain the limits of that promise. Patients must be informed and parents reassured that confidentiality will be breached when the clinician learns that there is the potential for harm to self or others of the behaviors or choices reported by the adolescent patient. This provides broad latitude and requires judgment on the part of the physician concerning what constitutes "harm." The revelation that a 14-year-old patient has smoked some cigarettes or tried alcohol for the first time needs to be contrasted with the risks associated with that same patient having promiscuous unprotected sex. A clinician who believes that he has a trusting relationship with his patient may seek to counsel and intervene with the patient to modify a potentially risky behavior and seek to follow-up with the patient without informing a parent if the short-term risks are low and the patient is willing to change behavior. But, the threshold for breaching confidentiality is quite different for adult and adolescent patients. For adults, physicians are obligated not to breach confidentiality unless there is clear evidence that the patient intends to harm himself or others. On the other hand, adolescents are legitimately subject to parental supervision and guidance if they are part of a functional family, and clinicians have the duty to inform parents if their child is in danger. The problem for the clinician is determining if revealing the information to a parent might result in the child being subject to abuse or abandonment. In such cases, the clinician may seek the support of a child-protection agency, but should not take it upon him- or herself to deal with the problem without informing another responsible person. If the clinician has decided that he must breach confidentiality and inform his patient's parent, he has a clear obligation to explain the basis of this decision to the patient. It is often helpful to do this conversation with the patient and parent together in the office, rather than by phone call to the parent. This allows the patient to feel a bit more protected as a plan for resolution of the problem is discussed.

THE ADOLESCENT ALONE

Most adolescents live at home in families that are more or less supportive and nurturing. But there are many young people who are isolated and separated from their families. Adolescents who are unsupervised because of being in dysfunctional or homeless families, or completely alone because of being orphans, runaways, throwaways, or street kids, are basically left without support or guidance from a caring adult. These youngsters often come in contact with the healthcare establishment because of serious medical and psychological problems. They rarely seek help until there are urgent and significant issues to address. They sometimes are arrested or found on the street and brought to hospital emergency departments for care. The adolescent alone can present particularly problematic issues for clinicians who wish to help them.

Although all adolescents are in various stages in the process of developing their own identities and capabilities in order to function as adults, many of the adolescents who are alone may seem to be more mature than their more mundane counterparts who live in nurturing families, but this apparent maturity may actually only be a superficial and a shrewd adaptation to the hazards of a very precarious existence. The adolescent alone is far more likely to be cognitively impaired and to be engaging in serious risk-taking behaviors including promiscuous sexual activity, illegal drug use, and stealing, as well as to be suffering from mental illness, malnutrition, sexually transmitted diseases, and a myriad of unaddressed chronic disorders. Some adolescents are accompanied to healthcare visits by adults who claim to be interested and responsible for the young person. These adults often have no legal guardianship or even a continuous relationship with the child. They are sometimes involved with the teens as pimps or drug dealers or in otherwise exploitative relationships for their own personal gain.

The adolescent alone has a very ambiguous legal status that can create some major problems related to consent for treatment and the maintenance of confidentiality. There are provisions in the laws of most states that will permit healthcare professionals to treat these young patients without involving parents or reporting them to child-protection agencies. The mature-minor doctrine and specific medical consent laws for sexually transmitted disease, reproductive health, pregnancy, drug and alcohol abuse, and mental health may allow clinicians to address some of the needs of these patients, but there is often no stable environment in which the youngster can recuperate after treatment, store medications, and seek support, and there is often no source to pay for the care and treatment.

Because of all of the complexity and ambiguity of entering into a clinical relationship with an adolescent alone, some pediatricians may not wish to care for these patients, but all clinicians should be aware of receptive programs and clinics where such young people may be referred for treatment. These programs and the professionals who staff them need to keep in mind several important ethical issues. First, clinicians have an ethical responsibility to treat these patients with respect, and to assist them to make reasonable choices about their care. All adolescents are in the process of becoming autonomous and are developing the capacity to make decisions in their own interest. This process requires the help of trusted adults, but these teens may be less trusting of adults and will need to develop trust over time with healthcare professionals. Keeping this in mind, clinicians will need to consider alternative approaches to treatment that are not threatening to the patient, that minimize the potential for harm, that are consistent with the patient's social reality, and that engage the patient in the decision each step of the way. Visit times may need to be flexible, medications may need to be stored at the clinic, counseling sessions may need to be brief and nonjudgmental, and harm-reduction strategies to reduce risky behaviors may be more appropriate than attempts at completely eliminating the risks.

Clinicians should not think of themselves as parents of these young-sters but, rather, as counselors whose beneficence-based obligations include attempting to promote the well-being of their patients. Health professionals will often be disappointed and frustrated by these patients, and will need to respond as clinicians, not parents, utilizing skills in mediation and compromise. Because the world of an adolescent alone is so dangerous and frightening, clinicians should work with the patient to consider options for identifying a safe, supportive, and responsible adult or program that can assist them in making decisions about their future. This is especially important if the teen has a chronic medical or mental health illness that will require ongoing treatment. Some patients will not be able to find an ongoing supportive person in their lives, but clinicians should continue to advocate for the adolescent to find a program that can be helpful.

Adolescents alone may refuse recommended treatments or counseling and may vote with their feet and not return for scheduled visits. In the face of a life-threatening emergency, refusal of treatment creates a seri-ous ethical concern for clinicians. Autonomous adults are permitted to refuse any medical interventions even when the provider believes it is not in the patient's interest to refuse. Many adolescents alone will have the capacity to make autonomous choices, but refusal of an acutely needed life-sustaining treatment in such a patient should not be met initially with acceptance. If possible, refusal should result in an extended period of discussion, clarifying the medical facts and consequences, exploring the reasons for refusal, eliminating barriers to acceptance of treatment, and examining any alternative treatments. Coercion or the use of force should rarely, if ever, be considered. If there remains a question about the young person's capacity, then attempts should be made to ensure that treatment is provided, but if the teen is deemed to have capacity and does not reverse his choice, ultimately his refusal of treatment should prevail. If the adoles-cent has a chronic and, likely, terminal disease, issues of resuscitation and continuing treatment should be discussed prospectively and plans made consistent with the teen's values and beliefs.

In the case of the adolescent alone, clinicians have the obligation to maintain confidentiality as would be the case in their relationships with other adolescents. Healthcare professionals should assure the young per-son that confidentiality will be protected except in certain, limited circum-stances. If such a limited circumstance should arise, like the commission of a criminal act, or the revelation that the teen is about to harm himself or others, the clinician should assure the teen that he will be informed about who will be told and what will be disclosed. Most important, in the case of an adolescent alone, the clinician should assure the patient of their willingness to continue to treat and support the young person and not abandon him even if the police or the courts are involved.

HOMOSEXUAL AND TRANSGENDER ISSUES

Adolescence is certainly a time of psychological turmoil, much of it associated with sexual experimentation and the development of sexual orientation and gender identity. Pediatricians need to get a broad understanding of their adolescent patients by asking about many aspects of their lives including questions about home life, school, what they do each day and on the weekends, their use of drugs and alcohol, thoughts and acts related to sexuality, and feelings of depression. Clinicians are often questioned by adolescent patients about sexuality, and particularly about whether the teen may be homosexual because of feelings of sexual attraction to members of the same sex. There are very few places where teens feel free to raise these issues, and pediatricians need to set a tone of openness to encourage patients to discuss sexuality and to answer any questions that may arise. A policy of privacy and respect for confidentiality is a needed prerequisite to such open discussions. In addition, asking questions based on the physical and emotional development of the teen, about onset of menstruation, sexual arousal, masturbation, sexual encounters and experience can be very important.

An older adolescent who only has persistent sexual and emotional attraction to persons of their own gender and has experimented with sexual activity with someone of their own gender, may be homosexual; but pediatricians should be aware there is much variability in sexual feelings and actions during adolescence. Clinicians should validate these sexual feelings and experiences as normal, natural, and acceptable, but should not be in a hurry to use a label to describe them. Questioning the teen in a nonjudgmental manner about the circumstances of the sexual encounter, the age of the partner, and their feelings afterward are important. It is the clinician's responsibility to ensure that such sexual encounters were consensual and not part of abuse or exploitation of the adolescent.

When an adolescent feels certain that he or she is homosexual and wishes to reveal this fact to their parents and family, the clinician should be available to participate in that conversation and facilitate communication among the participants. The coming-out process is an individual experience for each teen. Disclosing their status to friends, teachers, clergy, and others can be extraordinarily stressful and may require the help of a counselor well versed in these issues. Pediatricians should keep in mind that homosexual teens are susceptible to significant depression and that there is an increased incidence of suicide in this population. In addition, some families are not accepting of homosexual children and may shun them, physically abuse them, and throw them out of their homes. Clinicians should have information available about shelters and programs for homosexual teens if needed.

Some adolescents voice concerns about their biologic gender itself. Although sexual orientation relates to an individual's pattern of physical and emotional attraction to others, gender identity is an individual's internal sense of being male or female. A teenage boy's sexual orientation may be physical attraction only to other males, but his gender identity, based on his internal sense, may be either male or female. When an individual's biologic sex and gender identity are not in agreement, they are generally referred to as transgender, regardless of biologic sex or sexual orientation. The term transsexual is used for individuals who are transgender and seek to change (or have changed) their physical characteristics to match their inner sense of gender identity.

A young teen or even younger child may reveal a sense of alienation to some or all of the physical characteristics or social roles of their assigned biologic gender. This clinical manifestation is called gender dysphoria. Those children with gender dysphoria, who through alterations in behavior or appearance seek to resemble characteristics of the gender opposite to their biologic one, are deemed to be gender nonconforming. Gender nonconforming behavior is quite common in young children and early adolescents and should not be confused with or labeled as homosexuality. A young adolescent girl may wish to behave or dress like a boy, and at the same time develop physical and emotional attraction to boys. Children who early in life indicate that they "are," rather than "wish to be," a gender different from their biologic sex, and continually express concern about the difference between their physical sex and their gender identity, are more likely to evolve into a transgender adolescent. Children and adolescents who exhibit persistent and significant gender nonconforming behavior may benefit from a mental health counselor with experience in this area. Such therapy should not be focused on reversing or mediating gender dysphoria or attempting to change gender nonconforming behavior but, rather, should provide needed social support to the young person, and at the same time help the teen understand their complex feelings and cope with them. Many young children do not persist with gender noncon-forming behaviors into their teen years, and only 15–25% of adolescents who present to gender identity clinics show persistence of significant gen-der dysphoria into adulthood. It is important to note that many of these adults who experienced gender dysphoria in childhood identify as homo-sexual, but do not wish to pursue the path of transsexuality.

This field of medicine is relatively new, and there are few research stud-ies to support the recommendations of experts. But there are some basic ethical considerations that can guide efforts to help these young people. Each person should be allowed and encouraged to express his or her own sexual identity and to make choices consistent with those beliefs and feel-ings. Sexual orientation may be innate, but it is not immutable, it is fluid and evolves over time. Thus, clinicians need to refrain from inappropriate labeling, be accepting of their patient's concerns, and be nonjudgmental in their counseling. Some clinicians may not accept differences in sexual orientation or gender identity as a normal part of the human condition. But these clinicians should not impose those views on their patients and should find other more accepting physicians to care for these patients. Pediatricians need to help young persons develop their ability to make choices about all aspects of their futures, not by imposing personal or per-ceived societal values on them, but by helping them to develop positive identities regardless of their choices. Physicians can also play an impor-tant role in developing societal acceptance of individuals with varying sexual identities and work to decrease stigma and discrimination.

Perhaps the most ethically vexing aspect of caring for transgender youth is the decision about medical intervention to prepare for the ultimate physi-cal transition to the desired sex. Pediatricians should refer such youth to special programs in academic medical centers with experience and expertise caring for young transsexual patients. A team of endocrinologists, surgeons, psychiatrists, and psychologists is needed to help patients accomplish their goals. Endocrinologists can provide hormonal treatment to suppress endog-enous pubertal development and promote cross-gender secondary sexual characteristics. These medical treatments are generally reversible without harm if stopped, but there are some potentially irreversible side effects that may occur. These include the possibility of suppressing the gonads to such an extent that they are unable to ever develop mature sperm or ova. A gender nonconforming adolescent who is considering the initiation of hormonal treatment to suppress pubertal development should be coun-seled and evaluated by a mental health professional with special expertise in these matters. Since hormonal treatment is a major therapeutic inter-vention, endocrinologists generally recommend that youth be considered for this treatment only if they demonstrate significantly increased gender dysphoria with the onset of puberty and the initiation of secondary sexual characteristics.

Consent to initiate hormonal treatment should be obtained from both the adolescent and his or her parents. If parents are uninvolved or unwilling to participate in the discussion or they refuse to consent, pediatric clinicians should generally defer treatment until the adolescent has reached the legal age of majority. This approach can be justified by the elective nature of the treatment, and the potential for irreversible harm if the teen changes his or her mind about moving forward with transsexuality. Hormonal treatment, over time, can assist the patient develop many of the secondary sexual characteristics of the desired gender. In addition to that transformation, some patients will wish surgical reconstruction to become physically consistent with their affirmed gender. There are multiple breast and genital surgical procedures available to accomplish these goals. Most experts require the patient to be an adult, above the age of majority, in order to proceed with surgery. This is ethically justified by the elective nature of the surgery and the major irreversible life altering nature of the procedures. Once an adult, the patient may consent for these procedures without involvement of parents or any other individuals.

MENTAL ILLNESS, DEPRESSION, AND SUICIDE

It is estimated that 20% of adolescents have a mental or behavioral health problem that would benefit from assessment and treatment. Illicit drug, marijuana, and alcohol use, family disruption including parental separation and divorce, depression, suicide, homicide, school violence, bullying, bipolar disorder, and schizophrenia are all common among adolescents. Pediatricians and other clinicians who care for adolescents are aware that there is an acute shortage of mental health professionals with interest, competence, and availability to treat teens. Clinicians who provide primary care to adolescents are perfectly situated to screen teens for mental, emotional, and behavioral health problems and to offer first-line counseling and treatments. This is particularly important for those patients who might not otherwise receive any mental health-care or receive help only after the problems become more severe. Many pediatric practices have hired or co-located mental health professionals in their office suites. This takes away much of the stigma, discomfort, and dislocation caused by referral to a mental health provider in a distant office, and it often makes both the patient and the parents more comfortable with accepting mental health care. The numbers of school-based mental health clinics have also increased as a strategy to remove barriers to accessing mental health services. Recent violence in schools have made communities more willing to pay for prevention services with the hope that the availability of mental health counselors within the school can identify and address problems that might otherwise result in catastrophic outcomes.

Pediatricians should integrate a brief psychosocial and mental health update into every acute-care and well-care visit. This should be accomplished routinely in confidence with the patient, and annually with the parent, to assess how the young person is functioning at home, with friends, and at school. Signs of dysfunction, isolation, depression, poor school performance, and drug and alcohol use can be noted, and initial counseling provided. Reinforcing healthy lifestyles concerning nutrition, exercise, smoking, alcohol, screen time, stress management, and promotion of social interactions can be helpful, and follow-up visits to assess progress are essential. At times, referral to a social worker, psychologist, psychiatrist or psycho-pharmacologist may be needed.

Suicide is the third most common cause of death in adolescents, responsible for over 4000 deaths per year in the Untied States. It is likely that this is an underestimate of the actual number of deaths from suicide since many deaths reported as accidents, homicides, and drunk driving in youths are in fact suicides. Suicide attempts also cause significant morbidity, functional loss, and disability among those who attempt to kill themselves, and often injure others who are inadvertently affected. Since up to 90% of adolescents who commit suicide have a diagnosable psychiatric disorder at the time of death and more than half have had significant symptoms for longer than two years, this important cause of death and disability among youth is clearly amenable to primary prevention. In addition, approximately one-third of suicide victims have made a previous suicide attempt, making secondary prevention possible. National representative samples of United States high school students in grades 9 through 12 consistently report that 20–25% have seriously considered attempting suicide in the past 12 months, 15–18% have made a plan, and 8–10% have made an attempt.

Perhaps the most important factor in the successful accomplishment of suicide is the availability of a lethal means of self-harm. Firearms are the leading cause of death for both males and females who commit suicide, and over 60% of all suicides in youth in the United States are by firearms. Close to 50% of households in the United States have a firearm, and adolescents who commit suicide are most often not those who purchased the weapon. The availability of a gun in the home, regardless of whether it is kept unloaded or stored in a locked cabinet, is directly correlated with successful suicide.

Pediatricians can play a key role in the prevention of suicide in adolescents. Parental knowledge of their adolescent's feelings and behaviors is significantly limited and may be affected by the natural separation between parent and child that occurs during this period. Pediatricians should be assessing whether their patient appears isolated, depressed, has low self-esteem, or expresses any suicidal thoughts or behaviors. The pediatrician's office rather than a mental health facility may be viewed by the teen as a more acceptable place for initial discussion and evaluation of such symptoms.

Each teen should be asked at least annually: "Have you ever felt so unhappy that you wished you were dead?" If answered affirmatively, it can be followed by questions concerning thoughts about killing oneself, plans (method, time, and place), the availability of means (guns, pills, etc.), and any previous attempts, regardless of whether discovered or not. There is no evidence that asking an adolescent about suicidal ideation and assessing suicidal intent will precipitate the behavior. Conversely, raising these issues may be met with feelings of relief and can be reassuring to the teen to learn that someone will intervene to help them.

Confidentiality should be breached whenever adolescents are clearly at risk of hurting themselves or others. If the patient describes behaviors or feelings that suggest a significant risk of attempting suicide, the pediatrician should explain that he will not allow the teen to hurt him or her self and that they must involve others in creating a plan to help. This plan should undoubtedly include informing the parents. Parents are often unwilling to accept the seriousness of a report of suicidal ideation or recognition of early at-risk symptoms, and may be reluctant to seek mental health intervention for their child. The pediatrician must be firm and make clear recommendations about the situation. The stigma associated with the diagnosis of mental illness and the fear of referral for treatment must be addressed. Hospitalization for evaluation and the development of a treatment plan may be indicated. Because many general pediatric or adolescent medical units are inadequate for this purpose, the pediatrician in consultation with an adolescent psychiatrist or other qualified mental health professional should determine the optimal environment for the teen. A plan for immediate referral to an experienced mental health professional without hospitalization may be adequate in specific cases, but in the instance of a serious suicide attempt, hospitalization should be the norm.

From an ethical perspective, involuntary hospitalization is appropriate and justified for a teenager who has attempted suicide. The refusal of the young person to accept hospitalization should not be respected. A serious attempt to take one's own life is justification enough to override the autonomy of any patient. A brief hospital stay can be important to assess the level of mental illness in the patient, the likelihood of recurrence, and the need for medication, and to develop of a plan for follow-up. The hospital stay also provides a time to address any parental ambivalence about recognizing the seriousness of the situation, and to engage the family in the treatment and follow-up plan.

Pediatricians also play an important role in dealing with a child who has made an unsuccessful attempt at suicide. Fewer than 50% of adolescents who attempt suicide are referred for mental health evaluation or follow-up, and a large percent of those who are referred never follow through with appointments. No attempt at self-destructive behavior should be trivialized although some are much less serious than others. Most suicide attempts come to the attention of a general pediatrician or an emergency room physician. Pediatricians can evaluate the seriousness of the attempt and insist that, if the child does not require hospitalization, the teen should be fully evaluated and referred for immediate mental health follow-up. Referral should be accompanied by discussion with the family about the seriousness of this event and obtaining a commitment that they will follow through with the evaluation and treatment.

In any case in which suicide ideation or an attempt has occurred and even in cases in which adolescents merely reveal mood disorders, impulsive behaviors, or depressive symptomatology without a suicide attempt, pediatricians must address the potential danger of having a gun in the home. Pediatricians are generally encouraged to incorporate questions about gun ownership into history taking and urge parents who possess guns to remove them from the home. In the case of an adolescent who is at risk for suicide, this is an essential part of the management plan. Although some parents believe guns are an important part of recreational activities or are critical to the protection of the well-being of their family, parents faced with an adolescent at risk for suicide must recognize the substantial danger of any gun in the home. Even guns locked in closed cabinets can be the means for an adolescent intent on suicide.

EATING DISORDERS

Eating disorders, anorexia nervosa and bulimia, are increasing in the United States in both males and females of all ethnic and racial groups. Approximately 2% of adolescents suffer from an eating disorder. Girls are far more common than boys to suffer from these disorders, but about 10% of all eating disorders occur in males. Anorexia nervosa is a disorder in which the patient refuses to maintain body weight at or above a minimal level for age and height. This is generally associated with an intense fear of gaining weight although the individual is underweight and with a psychological disturbance in the way that body weight or shape is experienced. Bulimia is a disorder involving recurrent, frequent episodes of binge eating associated with inappropriate compensatory behaviors to prevent weight gain such as vomiting, use of laxatives, diuretics, enemas, or excessive exercise. There appears to be a family predisposition to eating disorders, and a genetic association with various common traits including perfectionism, behavioral rigidity, and harm avoidance.

Dieting, concern with body image and shape, and excessive exercise are common among many adolescents who wish to emulate supermodels, athletes, and movie stars, and voice the belief that "you can't be too thin." This societal emphasis on body image reflected in films and magazines has been implicated as a potent risk factor for the development of an eating disorder. Adolescents with eating disorders who become severely underweight are likely to suffer from significant complications and even death. Amenorrhea and menstrual irregularities are often first signs of an eating disorder in girls. Dehydration electrolyte abnormalities, inability to maintain body temperature, endocrine abnormalities, arrhythmias, and severe constipation are often later problems that precede collapse or even death.

Pediatricians need to be cognizant of these disorders, obtain routine vital signs including weight and height at least annually, question their patients about recent weight loss, and assess menstrual status regularly. If an eating disorder is suspected, clinicians can ask the patient whether they believe they are too thin, whether food dominates their thinking, whether they make themselves sick when they feel full, and whether they believe they have lost weight over the last few months. There are many causes of weight loss. Pediatricians should be diligent in evaluating a patient with a suspected eating disorder to rule out other treatable medical conditions such as gastrointestinal, oncologic, and endocrine diseases that can result in similar findings.

When the diagnosis of an eating disorder is confirmed, a multidisciplinary team including a physician, nutritionist, and mental health professional with expertise in these disorders is required to treat the problem. A treatment plan to prevent further weight loss and to create minimum weight goals is needed. Involvement of the adolescent is critical to the long-term success of the treatment. Intensive out patient treatment is needed, including frequent visits to the mental health professional. The patient needs to be engaged in the treatment plan from the beginning. Parents play an important role in assuring that the patient is eating and that any abnormal behaviors such as vomiting or excessive exercise are minimized. Day treatment programs and in-patient hospitalization may be required when weight loss is so profound that it seriously jeopardizes the young person's health. A patient's refusal to acknowledge that she or he is ill or unwillingness to agree to comply with the treatment plan or attend necessary appointments should result in an immediate response from the treatment team and the family. Here, again, the adolescent's autonomy cannot be respected because of the harmful consequences that may ensue. The treatment team must make clear to the patient that they will not allow her to hurt herself and risk death or disability from this disorder. Involuntary hospitalization, psychotropic drugs, and tube feeding, if necessary, may be needed to reverse the downward spiral of weight loss that jeopardizes the life and health of the teen.

Once the patient's body weight and weight gain are stabilized, the adolescent can gradually regain responsibility for their eating behavior and address any psychological issues that need resolution to ensure against recurrence. Reversal of the acute weight loss caused by an eating disorder is often accomplished, but many young people are susceptible to recurrence of weight loss and the pathologic behaviors that were associated with the problem; there are also high rates of long-term mental health issues including depression, anxiety, and obsessive behaviors that persist after the weight loss is resolved.

FINAL THOUGHTS

Adolescence is an extraordinarily important period in the life of any child. It is a time of profound biologic, psychologic and social development, and the gateway to adulthood. From an ethical perspective, we should respect and nurture the evolving autonomy of the adolescent, while we accept that this young person will undoubtedly benefit from our support and may need protection from impulsive and harmful behaviors. Adolescents who are critically and chronically ill are likely to have a keen sense of their personal preferences and values concerning treatment. Clinicians should keep these adolescents fully informed of their health status and of the available treatment options. Decision-making must include the adolescent as well as his or her parents, and pediatricians should generally support healthcare decisions made by older adolescents. Assessing the best interest of adolescents is challenging for families and clinicians alike, but critical for their successful transition to independent adult status.

ADDITIONAL READINGS

Alderman EM, Fleischman AR. Should adolescents make their own health care choices? *Contemp Pediatrics*, 1993; 10: 65–82.

Blustein J, Levine C, Dubler NN, eds. *The Adolescent Alone: Decision Making in Health Care in the United States*. New York, NY:Cambridge University Press; 1999.

Collogan LK, Fleischman AR. Adolescent research and parental permission. In: Kodish E, ed. *Ethics and Research with Children*. Oxford University Press, New York, NY: 2005: 77–99.

Fleischman AR, Barondess JA. Adolescent Suicide: vigilance and action to reduce the toll. *Contemp Pediatrics*, 2004; 21: 27–36.

A Hastings Center Special Report. *LGBT Bioethics: Visibility, Disparities, and Dialogue*. Powell T, Foglia MB, eds., New York, NY:*The Hastings Center Report*; 2014.

Rosen DS, and the American Academy of Pediatrics Committee on Adolescence. Identification and management of eating disorders in children and adolescents. *Pediatrics*, 2010; 126: 1240–1253.

Steever JB, Cooper-Server E. A Review of Gay, Lesbian, bisexual, and transgender youth issues for the pediatrician. *Pediatric Ann*, 2013; 42:2: 34–39.

Vance SR, Ehrensaft D, Rosenthal SM. Psychological and medical care of gender nonconforming youth. Pediatrics, 2014; 134: 1184–1189.

CHAPTER 9

Ethical Issues in Medical and Surgical Enhancement

Case 1

Bradley Parker is an 11-year-old boy who is 4 feet 1 inch tall. He and his parents, Susan and Harvey, have been referred to Dr. Debra Gartner, a pediatric endocrinologist at a large academic medical center for evaluation of short stature. Brad is quite concerned that he is the shortest boy in his class, does not do well in sports, and that the girls make fun of him and call him names like "Shorty." The referring pediatrician has noted that Brad's height had been at the fifth percentile, but his growth rate has slowed over the last two years. He has done some basic evaluations and decided it is time for Brad to be more fully evaluated. After a thorough history, physical exam, x-rays, and blood tests, Dr Gartner ascertains that Susan Parker is 5 feet 1 inches and Harvey Parker is 5 feet 7 inches tall; Brad is prepubertal and below the second percentile for height and at the twentieth percentile for weight. All endocrinologic and metabolic tests, including growth hormone stimulation tests are normal. Based on her findings, Dr. Gartner makes the diagnosis of idiopathic short stature and predicts that Brad's adult height will be about 5 feet 2 inches tall without treatment.

Case 2

Eric Spring is a 16-year-old high school student who was getting low grades and generally having difficulty in school. His mother brought him to see their family doctor, Dr. Paul Elias. Eric told Dr. Elias that he is disorganized, unable to focus on studying, inattentive in class, and often late in fulfilling school assignments. After a brief history suggesting that Paul had not had these types of problems in elementary and middle school, and that he appeared otherwise healthy, Dr. Elias administered a questionnaire and diagnosed Eric with attention deficit/hyperactivity disorder (ADHD), and prescribed a drug to enhance concentration and focus. Eric returned to see Dr. Paul after two weeks on treatment. He reported that the drug "jolted" him into being able to focus, and that he was able to study much better.

The desire to enhance human capacities and traits has existed since the beginning of the human race. Humans have sought to enhance their bodies so that they can run faster, grow taller, be stronger, and look better, and they have tried to enhance their minds so that they can accomplish more, be more empathic, appreciate the arts and music, and become more affluent, among other things. Parents generally wish to provide their children with opportunities to enhance their chances of success and optimize their potential. It is not surprising, then, that medicine has been asked to participate in the process of enhancing children. Modern medicine has within its armamentarium drugs to alter growth and modify mood, affect, and behavior, and surgical procedures to change many physical characteristics. And someday, medicine may be able to use the science of genomics through embryo selection or gene alteration to create enhanced capacities and the ability to choose desired traits. Do these types of enhancement activities fall within the fundamental goals of medicine? Should physicians be involved in fulfilling requests for enhancement of children?

The goals of medicine have often been described as the prevention and treatment of disease and the restoration of the patient to health and functionality. In this view, health is the absence of disease, suggesting that the goals of medicine should be construed narrowly as the prevention, treatment, and amelioration of disease. Most would agree to a somewhat broader definition of the goals of medicine to include maintenance of function, but few have argued that medicine should enhance human capability. Medicine, then, should attempt to ensure that people will have normal capacity and functionality in order to permit them to pursue those opportunities for which they are capable.

Although it may be understandable or even laudable for families to provide excellent nutrition, educational opportunities, music lessons, sports coaching, and various other exposures to enhance the performance or appearance of their children, it is not generally seen as the role of a physician to provide medical or surgical interventions that will make those same children have a competitive advantage or be able to extend their inherent capacities to fulfill their personal life goals. This view is also held by many health-policy experts who grapple with defining those minimal health interventions that should be provided to all children. They find the distinction between treatments that restore a patient to normal functionality and treatments that provide enhancement beyond normalcy to be helpful in determining which interventions should justly be included in insurance coverage and be part of the debates about basic benefits packages for universal access to health care.

In my opinion, the decision about whether it is ethical for physicians to provide medical or surgical enhancements to children should not be determined based on standards for the mandated minimum package of benefits provided by health-insurers. Insurers do not currently pay for everything that is within the purview of medicine. Some important treatments, such as growth hormone for idiopathic short stature in children, joint replacements for arthritis in elderly patients, or in vitro fertilization for infertile couples often are not part of health insurance coverage. These treatments are, nonetheless, viewed as ethically acceptable practices and have become an accepted part of the goals of medicine. Some might view growth hormone or artificial joints or infertility treatment as enhancements, but others view these interventions as providing important and meaningful benefits to various aspects of people's lives.

Those who argue that the goal of medicine is to restore the ill to normal health ignore the impact of that view on individuals who are disabled. Many people in our society who are disabled or appear different from the majority will never be able to be normal in the common meaning of that term. If the goal of medicine is solely to restore people to normalcy, doesn't this view devalue those who are different? Much of the suffering experienced by disabled or dysmorphic people is socially determined and value laden. If we glorify normalcy, we demean those who may not be able to or may not wish to fit into a socially constructed norm. We also inadvertently imply that those who wish voluntarily to remain different from the norm are less valued, and by doing so, we constrain their individual freedom. Having diversity in our midst should be valued, and assuming that the goal of medicine is to decrease that diversity and to create a more homogenous "normal" population may be harmful and inappropriate.

Another definition of health, from the perspective of the World Health Organization, is a "state of complete physical, mental, and social well being." In this ambitious view, the goals of medicine become far more expansive.

The definition implies that the goals of medicine are not merely to prevent or treat disease, but more broadly to affect those social determinants of health that account for much of our well-being. In this view, physicians are justified in providing medical or surgical interventions that seek to increase a patient's state of mental or social well-being beyond their inherent capability. If medicine might participate in enhancement, what are the circumstances in which this is ethically acceptable? The ethical issues and concerns in this area are complicated, require careful analysis, and, as is often the case, will differ based on context. It is important to review several common medical and surgical enhancement interventions in children in order to understand better the ethical complexity of these cases.

MEDICAL ENHANCEMENT

Pediatricians are regularly involved in providing medications that enhance their patients. The most common enhancements are the administration of a series of vaccinations to enhance the capacity of the immune system to prevent childhood diseases. This 20th-century public-health success story has saved the lives of countless children by creating a "new normal" ability on the part of a child's body to fight disease. In addition to immunizations, clinicians often prescribe vitamins, iron, and diet supplements to enhance nutrition, and drugs to increase the ability to concentrate or decrease anxiety and hyperactivity. Do children receiving these medications have a disease or disorder that requires treatment? Are there other appropriate interventions, short of providing medication that might be helpful to alleviate the problems or symptoms being addressed? Although some clinicians might call these approaches preventive interventions or treatments of disorders, for most children, these therapies are provided in response to concerned parents who wish to enhance their child's health, growth, or behavior. The nutritional supplements and the behavior modifying medications are often justified as optimizing the child's potential to grow, interact, learn, or perform on tests.

There are several common medical enhancements for children that deserve careful consideration and ethical analysis. These include growth hormone to enhance growth rate and ultimate adult height for children with idiopathic short stature, hormonal growth attenuation to enhance the quality of life of profoundly impaired children, drugs to modify the ability to concentrate and focus on learning for children with concentration and behavioral problems, and genetic engineering and embryo selection to choose desired traits for future children.

Growth Hormone for Idiopathic Short Stature

Short stature is one of the most common reasons for referral to a pediatric endocrinologist. Parents and children are concerned about the effect of being short on quality of life. A short child's difficulty in relating to peers, and poor ability at sports, as well as concern about ultimate height and its effect on various teen and adult capabilities, often motivate families to seek evaluation for remediable causes of short stature. Some children with short stature have genetic syndromes, and others are found to have growth hormone deficiency, hypothyroidism, or other metabolic and chronic diseases that are amenable to treatment. The vast majority of short children are diagnosed with idiopathic short stature. These children are generally healthy and have no clear evidence of an endocrinologic or genetic problem. By definition, children with idiopathic short stature have a height below the first percentile for age and sex. They generally have had a normal birth weight and gestational age and are growth-hormone sufficient. Approximately 500,000 children in the United States between the ages of 4 and 13 years are considered to have idiopathic short stature, many because of familial short stature, and others with a constitutional delay in growth and puberty.

Since the 1990s, recombinant human growth hormone has been available for treatment of children with short stature who have growth hormone deficiency. This drug, generally administered as subcutaneous injections on a daily basis for several years, has been shown to be effective, and there are national registries of treated patients to record any suspected side effects. In children with abnormally low levels of growth hormone, treatment will usually increase growth rate and ultimate adult height. Short-term risks of the drug are low, including headaches from increased intracranial pressure, glucose intolerance, and "growing pains" and slipped epiphyses at joints and jaw due to accelerated growth. There are no data on the potential long-term risks of cancer in adulthood because the drug has only been available for 25 years, but there is the possibility that there will be late epigenetic or direct affects on the incidence or severity of hormone-sensitive tumors.

Children with idiopathic short stature with normal levels of growth hormone secretion have been treated with exogenous growth hormone. These children often exhibit an increased growth rate, but only a 1–3 inch increase in adult height. The response is variable based on dose, age at onset of treatment, and genetic height potential. Many children with idiopathic short stature are treated with increasing doses of growth hormone in an effort to increase growth rate, resulting in an increased incidence of short-term side effects. The cost of treatment with growth hormone is currently about $30,000 per year. In 2003, the Food and Drug Administration approved the use of human growth hormone for children with idiopathic short stature, but most insurance companies will not pay for this treatment. Should pediatric endocrinologists prescribe human growth hormone for children with idiopathic short stature? Should short stature be considered a disability? Do the negative psychosocial consequences of being short warrant treatment that will only modestly increase adult height? Should insurance companies pay for this treatment? Should affluent families who can afford the cost of treatment be permitted to provide this enhancement to their children?

Bradley Parker, the 11-year-old boy in Case 1 in this chapter is diagnosed with idiopathic short stature by Dr. Gartner. Brad and his father, Harvey, are concerned that his height has caused Brad to be depressed and aloof. He is reluctant to participate in sports and has few friends. Dr. Gartner is impressed with the severity of these symptoms, but she is concerned that growth hormone may not do much to alleviate them. She explains the potential benefits of growth hormone, focusing on the short term acceleration of growth rate but makes sure that the family understands the likely modest increase in ultimate adult height for Brad. She also explains that some children benefit by a short-term increase in growth rate and are better able to participate in sports with their peers. Susan, Brad's mother, is most concerned about the predicted adult height of 5 foot 2 inches. Although she is only 5 foot 1 inch, she thinks that her height is more acceptable for a girl and will be difficult for a boy as a teen and young adult. She enjoys having a husband who is taller, and worries that girls will not be interested in Brad because of his height. She thinks that 2 to 3 inches of additional adult height could make a big difference in Brad's life.

Based on these conversations, Dr Gartner is willing to prescribe growth hormone for Brad, but she is sure, based on past experience, that the family's health insurance will not cover it. They all agree that Dr. Gartner should send all of the medical information to the insurance company and request approval for treatment. She asks the family to consider whether they can afford to pay for the treatment and agrees to see them again in a month.

Critical in the ethical analysis of growth hormone treatment for idiopathic short stature are the effects of short stature on young children and adolescents, the impact of being short on adults, and the benefits of such treatment weighed against the potential risks. Recent studies using health-related quality-of-life scales have revealed that short children and their parents concur that the children have lower emotional and social functioning, decreased self-esteem, and greater depressive symptoms than healthy peers. These findings improved after three months of treatment and were maintained over an additional 24 months of treatment. Older European studies suggest that there are few, if any, psychosocial problems in children whose height is below the third percentile in the general population. Not all children suffer negative psychosocial consequences of short stature and most short adults report no increase in psychosocial problems.

I believe that pediatricians are justified in prescribing human growth hormone for selected patients with idiopathic short stature. It should be noted that some of these patients may be found in the future to have a physiological abnormality, not just a constitutional one, as further knowledge is gained from research. Having a normal level of growth hormone may not be the only determinant of growth rate and height. If new disorders are identified, those short children will have lost the opportunity to be treated for their abnormality. Nonetheless, there should be specific criteria for treatment of idiopathic short stature, including: height below the first percentile for sex and age, a clear indication from the child of significant negative psychosocial impact from being short, and a willingness on the part of child and parents to be followed longitudinally and to participate anonymously in the national registry. I am in agreement with Dr. Gartner in our case, but I believe that individual pediatric endocrinologists are justified in conscientiously objecting to treatment of idiopathic short stature based on the impression that there is no disease or physiological abnormality present, and/or that there is only modest benefit of the treatment in such cases. Physicians who conscientiously object to prescribing growth hormone in these circumstances should inform the family of the diagnosis, counsel them about the risks and benefits of treatment, and make a recommendation against treatment because they believe the benefits of treatment are not sufficient to outweigh the risks. In addition, they should inform the family that other physicians may have a different view and may be willing to provide the treatment.

Some endocrinologists who oppose treatment of idiopathic short stature with growth hormone believe that it is inappropriate to treat socially constructed problems with medications. They argue that even if short children have problems in psychosocial functioning, it is not because of their physical status but because of attitudes and behaviors of individuals in the society in which we live. They believe interventions should focus on changing height prejudice and the attitudes and behaviors of others toward short people, as well as on making reasonable adaptations for short people in public spaces, not on changing the inherent characteristics of the victims of this discrimination. Other clinicians note that medicalizing the problem of short stature in an otherwise healthy child by testing, daily injections, and continual care, runs the risk of worsening the psychological impact of being short on the child rather than improving it.

Another important aspect of this treatment is the cost. Even though growth hormone is approved for this indication, most insurance companies will not pay for the drug for these children. Few families can afford $20,000–$50,000 per year for several years of treatment. Because those who are less well off will be unable to afford the drug, should we preclude the affluent from obtaining it? I think not. We should only prevent use of the drug if it is harmful. Since the psychological symptoms associated with short stature appear significant, at least in some patients, and the treatment has some level of efficacy and a reasonable safety record to date, we should not argue that withholding this treatment from an individual child is in that child's best interest. The assessment of best interest and the ultimate decision should be left to the child and family.

Some have argued that the cost is so high that if we prescribe growth hormone and allow affluent families to pay for it, resources will be diverted from other important healthcare needs. This is just not the case. Affluent families can choose to send their children to private schools, may buy them expensive cars, and take them on luxurious trips, but that does not, in and of itself, divert resources from needed programs for poor children. Buying the drug for an affluent child does not deprive others of needed treatments or programs. It is certainly unfair that some families who believe it is in their child's best interest to have the treatment will be deprived of that option because of cost; but that circumstance is not unique to this situation. In many countries the decision is made nationally about which children are eligible to receive growth hormone, or other expensive treatments, regardless of socioeconomic status. That is not the case in the United States. Our country has chosen to allow inequities in healthcare access, quality, and treatment. It should be noted that in countries where growth hormone is not available to affluent children with idiopathic short stature, families often travel to the United States or one of several other countries where it can be prescribed by willing physicians and purchased for cash.

Although growth hormone for idiopathic short stature can be viewed as an enhancement that attempts to change the fundamental nature of a child who has no apparent physiological abnormality, I am sympathetic to the psychological and social problems experienced by short children. I believe this therapy is consistent with the goals of medicine that include the alleviation of suffering, and that the potential benefit, though modest, could make a real difference in the life of the child and future adult. This therapy should be offered to families with full and informed consent and without coercion, and prescribed for children whose family believes it is in the child's best interest.

Growth Attenuation in Children with Profound Developmental Disabilities

A family in Seattle several years ago had a six-year-old girl named Ashley who was bedridden, incontinent, and suffered from severe developmental disabilities. They wished to care for Ashley at home, but feared that she would grow into an adolescent who would be hard to handle. Ashley was predicted to have an adult height of 5 feet 4 inches. Her parents requested that her doctors treat her with estrogen before her pubertal growth spurt to attenuate growth in order to enhance her future quality of life. Ashley's parents and her doctors justified this treatment by arguing that growth attenuation would result in Ashley having an adult height of approximately 4 feet 6 inches, which would allow her more easily to be cared for and to participate in family social and recreational activities inside and outside the home. Ashley's physicians were willing to provide this treatment. They sought the consultation of the hospital ethics committee who agreed that in Ashley's interest, as determined by her parents and their doctors, it was ethically justifiable to go forward with the growth attenuation plan.

Many individuals with severe disability, several advocacy groups, and many individual families of profoundly disabled children were infuriated by this treatment plan. They were very critical of the justification used to provide the treatment as enhancing the life of a disabled child. They argued that it is not in disabled children's interests to alter the natural growth of their bodies, and it is unethical to alter the bodies of children in order to advance the interests of their parents. Some also argued that society does not adequately accommodate to the needs of the disabled, and that this reality is no excuse for altering the bodies of the disabled in order to accommodate to the deficits of the society. Some families of adult disabled children were sympathetic to Ashley's parents and report that as their child grew to adult height and weight they were forced to greatly limit life experiences and recreational activities and had increasing problems with mobility, diaper changes and repositioning in bed. They saw growth attenuation as a creative solution to an inevitable problem that would allow profoundly disabled children to overcome the boredom and seclusion so common in this population.

I do not view growth attenuation in the context of a severely affected child as devaluing disabled children, and I do not believe that increasing resources for the care of the disabled, as laudable as that might be, can solve the problem of caring for profoundly disabled, severely cognitively impaired adolescents at home who have grown to a size that makes it difficult to manage their routine needs and to provide opportunities for social activities. When loving parents and competent physicians view a treatment plan that includes growth attenuation as in the best interest of a child like Ashley, I believe it should be implemented. It would be prudent to review the case with an ethics committee in order to ensure that there is transparency, broad agreement about the facts, and that the interest of the child is the primary motivator of the plan. It seems unnecessary and an excessive burden on the family to seek court approval for this treatment. Best interest assessments should be left to the parents in collaboration with their doctors, unless they are behaving in a manner that is clearly against the interests of the child. The fact that this treatment may offend some disability advocacy groups should not affect the decision, and should not be an excuse for seeking court approval of such treatments. Parents of chronically ill children make many healthcare decisions that have even more profound effects on the child's life without court intervention. Physicians and institutions should not prioritize concern about negative public opinion over family privacy and respect for parental discretion in decision-making for their children.

Psychotropic Drugs

Pediatricians are commonly asked to see young children and adolescents who are having trouble with school performance or behavior problems due to inability to concentrate, hyperactivity, or impulsivity. Parents and teachers alike want to enhance children's ability to concentrate and learn, and also want to decrease hyperactivity and impulsivity that impedes performance. Thousands of children each month are evaluated for attention deficit/hyperactivity disorder (ADHD), and most are placed on potent drugs to decrease symptomatology and improve performance. There are generally accepted criteria for the diagnosis of this disorder, but there is no specific blood test, genetic mutation, or metabolic marker that confirms the diagnosis. Since assessments of behavior are known to be subjective, clinicians are cautioned to obtain information not only from the child and family, but also from the school and other therapists involved in the child's care. It is estimated that 5–10% of young children and youths are diagnosed with ADHD and most are treated for several years. For those children with a serious problem that impairs their ability to learn, treatment is warranted and can enable them to enhance performance and fulfill their inherent potential.

Some critics of medicating children for hyperactivity argue that the increasing number of children on medication is a result of the failing educational system that cannot deal with normal variation in how children learn due to increasing class sizes and inexperienced teachers. They believe that children are naturally curious, have short attention spans, and need creative and individualized approaches to maintain their interest in learning. Critics blame teachers for insisting that children be evaluated for hyperactivity because they are unwilling to put in the effort required to teach children of various capabilities. There is no question that some of the children currently on medication for ADHD are misdiagnosed and are being medicated unnecessarily. Some of these children are not able to learn in the classroom because of cognitive impairment or mental health disorders other than ADHD. Other children do not require medication to learn but might need more individualized educational opportunities.

I do not believe we should view treatment for ADHD as enhancement. These medications, when prescribed appropriately for the right patients, are potentially effective therapies for a serious disorder, not an attempt to enhance the ability of a child to learn beyond their inherent potential. I do not believe that most parents who seek care for children who are having problems learning seek treatment to enhance their child's ability to learn above what is his or her potential. Nonetheless, there are too many children who are being diagnosed and treated for ADHD. This remains an important issue in pediatrics and requires physicians and psychologists to be careful about labeling a child with this diagnosis and prescribing potent medications for children who will not benefit from them.

There is another group of young people who have not experienced ADHD as a child, but have heard from their parents, friends, or the media that they can increase their ability to succeed in school by taking drugs that enhance concentration. Eric Spring, the 16-year-old boy in Case 2 in this chapter, was enjoying goofing off in high school, not studying, and getting drunk with this friends in the town park on the weekends. His grades were very poor and his parents were concerned. The school guidance counselor explained to Eric that he was in jeopardy of being left back if he did not complete assignments and pass all his final exams this semester. Eric heard from some friends that if he was cool and said the right things, he could convince his doctor to prescribe a drug that would give him a great high, and at the same time help him complete schoolwork and study for exams. Eric told his parents that his teachers recommended that he see his doctor to get some medicine to help with paying attention in school. Eric's mother brought him to see Dr. Elias, asking for help with concentration. Dr. Elias did not learn much from Mrs. Spring about Eric's symptoms, and he did not get records from the school or call the guidance counselor. He prescribed a potent drug in an attempt to enhance concentration without taking into account the context of the patient's problem.

Psychotropic drugs for enhancing school performance can be dangerous. They can cause overstimulation, insomnia, weight loss, depression, palpitations, hypertension, psychotic symptomatology, and even sudden death. These drugs are controlled substances because they have been abused, resulting in extreme psychological dependence. It is hard to ethically justify the use of psychotropic drugs to enhance concentration in adolescents without a clear diagnosis of ADHD and careful monitoring and follow up. It is also ethically questionable whether drugs should be used for this purpose when behavioral interventions are available to help students learn how to organize work, study, and enhance test taking performance.

Embryo Selection and Genetic Engineering

When embryos are produced through in vitro fertilization, preimplantation genetic diagnosis (PGD) may be performed to ascertain the sex of the embryo and whether it has a chromosomal or genetic disorder. This technique (discussed at some length in chapter 2, Ethical Issues in Creating a Child) will have the potential in the near future to screen embryos for desirable and undesirable traits associated with particular genes. PGD seems easily justifiable for embryo selection for cases in which serious chromosomal or genetic disorders are suspected. The more controversial uses of PGD include selecting for unwanted or wanted traits that are genetically determined. This practice permits consideration of negative and positive eugenics, improvement of humanity through the elimination or, at least, reduction of the number of individuals with unwanted characteristics, and the increase of persons with desired traits. Few of the most likely traits of interest—such as intelligence, height, longevity, or physical strength and prowess—are determined by a single or even a small number of genes that could be assessed using PGD. But it is certainly possible that, as the science of genomics progresses, genetic determinants of various traits that might be of interest to prospective parents will be found. Embryos with nondesired traits could then be destroyed or genetically engineered to alter those traits. Should PGD and genetic engineering be used for eugenics? Should future parents select those embryos that have the highest likelihood of producing children with the "best" possible lives?

There are countries, like England, Germany, and Italy, where medical practices in reproductive technologies are highly regulated. Governmental organizations determine which procedures will be permitted and clinicians are obligated to comply with these regulations. In the United States, we believe that individuals and their physicians have a broad range of procreative liberty. Although quite controversial, couples are permitted to create and destroy embryos, decide whether they wish to continue a pregnancy or terminate it, and have had wide latitude in obtaining genetic information about their future child through prenatal and intrauterine testing. PGD is just one part of this procreative freedom. United States law permits couples to practice eugenics through the use of PGD, but the more important question is this: should couples be permitted to use PGD to choose a future child with characteristics that they find appealing? And, should clinicians provide the needed knowledge and skills to permit this to be successful? I believe parents will demand PGD for eugenic purposes as soon as such testing becomes possible and available. I also believe that there will be infertility programs that will readily provide these services.

Parents have always wished to enhance the chances of their children being born healthy and leading productive lives. Pregnant women ought to be permitted to obtain knowledge about their prospective child's health and well-being and to decide whether or not to reproduce. However, regardless of the genetic information obtained from PGD, it would be naïve for parents to believe that genetic information alone will determine their child's ultimate outcome. It will remain very difficult, even with increasingly specific genetic information, to determine those embryos that have the highest likelihood of producing children who will have the best possible lives.

Are there potential harms to the future child or to others in society of parents learning about nonmedically related characteristics of their child and then deciding whether to proceed with the pregnancy? If an embryo is destroyed or a pregnancy terminated, the child who would have been born will never exist. If one believes that an embryo or fetus has significant moral status, it is easy to argue that by destroying the child who would have been born he or she is harmed. On the other hand, if an embryo or fetus has no or little inherent moral status, there is no future person who is being harmed by not gestating that particular embryo or fetus. I share this latter view.

However, it is possible to argue that others in society will be harmed by widespread use of PGD for eugenic purposes. Some commentators believe that reproduction is a natural lottery, and prospective parents should not attempt to change the natural process of procreation by altering the children who are destined to be born. Doing so hurts the richness and diversity of our society. Some individuals with genetic disorders and many people with disabilities argue that PGD and embryo selection denigrates those who are disabled or suffer from inherited diseases. Some advocates for patients with rare genetic disorders believe that having the ability to prevent the birth of children with these disorders harms those already born with the disorders by decreasing interest and investment in developing therapeutic interventions. Another harmful effect of the use of PGD for embryo selection will be the inequitable availability of this technology and the potential for a disproportionate incidence of negative traits in minority or impoverished populations. This unfairness has been part of the use of the new reproductive technologies since its inception and will continue as long as all private and public insurers do not pay for these procedures.

I believe the field of reproductive endocrinology, led by its national associations, ought to resist the widespread use of PGD to screen all embryos for eugenic purposes and non-health-related enhancements of future children. PGD is appropriately used for couples who are at risk for creating a fetus with a serious genetic disorder because of their known carrier status. As PGD becomes more available, it will be important to set professional standards that strongly discourage clinicians from participating in broad based eugenic and enhancement practices, and criticize those who do.

SURGICAL ENHANCEMENT

Cosmetic surgery in adolescents, particularly on the nose, has been performed with the consent of the child and parents for decades. Many teens wish to alter their inherent facial features in an attempt to enhance attractiveness. They often want to complete these cosmetic procedures before ending high school and embarking on college, which means they will be below the legal age of majority in most cases. Although I am not in favor of changing an adolescent's face without a medical or health-related reason, I can understand why some teens and young adults might wish to enhance their appearance with facial surgery. This type of enhancement has become standard practice for those who want it and can afford it. Operations on the nose have significant risks associated with anesthesia, airway compromise, bleeding, and postoperative complications. I think it would be impossible to reverse this practice and prevent teens from obtaining this type of surgical enhancement, but individual surgeons are justified in not performing these procedures on adolescents who have not reached the age of majority. The risks and irreversible nature of surgical interventions, along with the preoccupation of teens with their appearance and the need to be liked by peers, makes the informed-consent process more complex and difficult. The physician should spend sufficient time with the patient to be assured that the young person is serious about wanting the surgery, has considered the option of waiting, and understands the possible complications, before obtaining consent. Parents should be involved in these decisions for teens and their permission should be mandatory for this completely optional and elective procedure.

Adolescent patients are increasingly requesting surgical interventions to change various aspects of their bodies. Breast augmentation and reduction, fat removal and sculpting of belly, thighs and buttocks, and facial reconstruction are among the most commonly requested enhancements. Many of the patients seeking these enhancements are young women who want to be models or actresses. Here again, physicians should be very careful about embarking on these surgical procedures with adolescent patients. Many of these patients are motivated by complex psychosocial concerns and run the risk of not being completely satisfied with the results of the surgery. Their disappointment may cause significant depression and even suicidal ideation. If the surgeon is willing, the young person and her parents need to be fully informed and committed to the surgery before embarking on this course of action.

There are two more complex surgical procedures to enhance children that are even more ethically problematic and require careful analysis: plastic surgery to change the facial characteristics of children with Down Syndrome, and extremity lengthening procedures for children with dwarfism.

Plastic Surgery in Down Syndrome

Down Syndrome is a genetic abnormality caused by an extra 21st chromosome. The syndrome includes characteristic facial features, delayed development, cognitive impairment, moderate short stature, and is often associated with anatomic abnormalities of the heart and bowel. Over the last several decades, the potential for higher cognitive and social functioning among children with Down Syndrome has been appreciated, and early intervention programs, mainstreaming programs in schools, and fostering interaction between children with Down Syndrome and average children have resulted in increasing cognitive capability, and enhancing self-esteem, peer acceptance, and social functioning in these children.

Most parents of children with Down Syndrome are committed advocates, seeking to enhance the cognitive and social abilities of their children. Nutritional supplements, exercise programs, hormonal treatments, antidementia medicines, and alternative and complementary therapies have all been used with variable success. There are some ethical concerns about these approaches because this population and their parents are vulnerable to exploitation, and there are few clinical trials that confirm efficacy of these interventions. Clearly, more and better research is needed to define the efficacy and complications of each of these therapies. However, attempts to normalize children with Down Syndrome are within the goals of medicine as applied to those who are disabled or cognitively impaired. These interventions are not attempting to enhance the children beyond what might be considered normal or average for their peers, but merely to help them optimize their potential.

A more controversial intervention for children with Down Syndrome is plastic surgery to change their facial features. The characteristic facial features of a child or adult with Down Syndrome are recognizable to most people and engender stereotypic assumptions related to cognitive capacity. Facial plastic surgery is justified as in the interest of the child because the enhanced appearance makes it less likely that the child will be recognized as having Down Syndrome. This could decrease the stigmatization associated with the diagnosis and might increase social acceptance. The surgery is also purported to improve physical functioning, because surgical intervention to decrease the size of the tongue can improve speech, diminish drooling, and make chewing and swallowing easier.

There have been several studies over the last 30 years concerning parental views on facial plastic surgery and its outcome. Studies that report results from parents who have consented to the surgery and from doctors who have performed it are overwhelmingly positive about outcome. Research using parents who have not been interested in the surgery for their own children but have observed it in others reveal far less positive results. Unfortunately, none of the studies include data from the children themselves.

A large study of parents of children with Down Syndrome suggests that although they are aware that such surgery exists, very few, perhaps only 1%, have subjected their children to these procedures. The overwhelming number of parents are opposed to the surgery because they accept their children, they don't wish to subject them to unrealistic expectations, and they are concerned about the pain and discomfort of the procedures. On the other hand, parents who are willing to consider facial surgery for their children believe it will alleviate social stigma, improve speech, and help their child to live a better life.

Research is clearly inconclusive about whether facial plastic surgery has any medical or psychological benefits for children with Down Syndrome. The social stigma associated with the diagnosis of Down Syndrome has decreased over the past decades, and most people have had the opportunity to interact with or at least to observe children with the disorder. Increasingly, studies have shown that social rejection of individuals who are different or have disabilities is associated with their behaviors, not their appearance; and there are no data to support an actual increase in social acceptance associated with altering the facial characteristics of children with Down Syndrome. We must question whether parents who wish to alter the facial appearance of their children with Down Syndrome are electing surgery in an effort to decrease their own negative perceptions about the disorder, and to satisfy their own needs, or to enhance the interests of their child. Should this surgery be permitted? Should facial surgeons agree to perform it? Should parents consider subjecting their child to the pain and discomfort of the surgery for the purported benefits?

I believe that currently our society is much more accepting of children with Down Syndrome than ever before, and willing to optimize their abilities and social interactions. Although we offer screening during pregnancy to identify fetuses with Down Syndrome, and permit termination of these pregnancies, we also increasingly accept children born with this disorder as full members of our community. Some have argued that any elective surgical interventions should be postponed until the young person is old enough to consent. In the case of cognitively impaired young people with Down Syndrome, waiting may not change their ability to provide full informed consent, and if the purported benefits are real, the surgery should probably take place fairly early in childhood. If parents request facial surgery, the views of the young person with Down Syndrome should be taken into account in deciding whether to operate. Their impressions about the procedure should be ascertained as best possible consistent with their developmental level and in a manner that does not frighten them.

Parents should be discouraged from facial surgery for children with Down Syndrome unless there is a clear medical reason such as difficulty breathing, speaking, or swallowing that would justify it. However, I do not believe that plastic surgery on children with Down Syndrome should be prohibited. If loving parents and their physicians agree that it is in the best interest of a specific child to have one of these procedures, I believe it should be permitted. I hope that if the procedure continues to be offered, research on the outcomes will be available, including a thorough examination of the thoughts and feelings of the children who are subjected to the surgery.

Limb Lengthening Surgery for Dwarfism

There are more than two hundred different genetic conditions that lead to dwarfism. About 1 in 25,000 children (or about 150 children per year in the United States) are born with Achondroplasia, the most common form of dwarfism representing about 75% of all dwarfs. Achondroplasia is an autosomal dominant genetic disease with 90% of the cases resulting from a fresh mutation. Normal couples discover through fetal ultrasound exams, or at birth, that their baby has short limbs, a normal torso and an abnormally large head. Children with Achondroplasia have normal organs, but may have problems with their necks and spines because of their large head and weak muscles. Learning to walk can be difficult and development of scoliosis is common. The average adult height of a woman with Achondroplasia is 4 feet, and a man is 4 feet 3 inches. Beginning in childhood, dwarfs are unable to function normally in a society that is made for taller people and for people with longer arms. Reaching things is a real problem and even wiping oneself after going to the bathroom is difficult.

Throughout the 20th century, orthopedic surgeons have developed techniques to lengthen the limbs of children with dwarfism as a method to enhance their ability to function in society. Limb lengthening has been considered both a cosmetic and a functional enhancement. Cosmetic because it allows the patient to be over a foot taller and much closer to average height, and functional because it enhances the ability of the person to take care of themselves and function within a society that is not very accommodating to people with short limbs. The actual limb lengthening procedure is a series of painful and complicated surgeries over a period of several years, commencing with the prepubertal growth spurt at about 8 to 10 years of age. After screws are inserted into the lower leg at one- to two-inch intervals, the bone is broken into about 10 pieces and the screws connected to an external brace for stability. Extending the brace moves the screws and permits the broken segments to be forced apart. After a few weeks, as the bone begins to heal, the brace is extended to stretch the broken segments again. This process is repeated until the bone is lengthened maximally consistent with stretching of the muscles and ligaments. After the lower legs, the lower arms are lengthened, and then the upper legs, and finally the upper arms. The children are forced to spend their preteen and early teen years in limb braces, suffering from painful procedures, and susceptible to significant surgical complications including bone infections and skin breakdown.

Many adults who have had limb-lengthening procedures believe it increases self- esteem, and is transformative in that it allows dwarfs to function normally in the society and to more easily interact with average people. But many advocates within the community of people with dwarfism oppose these procedures. They argue that their condition does not need to be corrected, and that parents must accept their child and help the child to accept him or herself. They believe that it is wrong to tell children that they will be "fixed," and then put them through such painful, perhaps barbaric, procedures.

Some families and some children can accept and even celebrate the uniqueness of being a dwarf, whereas others have great difficulty being different. Parents' attitudes and beliefs about their children directly affect how children feel about themselves, and parents' beliefs about limb lengthening will affect how children feel. It is possible for 8- or 9-year old children to voice their views about embarking on limb lengthening, but it is not possible for them to make an autonomous choice about this life-altering surgery. Unfortunately, the decision to begin the surgical procedures must be made during the active growth phase of childhood. It cannot be delayed until the child is old enough to make this decision for him or herself. Children with dwarfism and their families make a commitment to either embark on a journey that embraces difference or one that attempts to decrease difference and minimize disability. The surgical route can be viewed as both a step toward normalization and as an enhancement. It is an enhancement because it changes the very nature of the person and may alienate them from their authentic selves. Yet, I find the journey to overcome disability both a courageous and potentially rewarding one. I applaud both the families who choose to celebrate difference and those who seek to conquer it. From an ethical perspective, we need to be sure that both paths are available and that decisions are made with sufficient knowledge of the consequences of either route, because once the decision is made, it is virtually impossible to reverse the decision.

FINAL THOUGHTS

Parents will always want to help their children to be the very best that they can be, and we should permit and even encourage families to optimize their child's inherent potential. But there may come a time when science will enable parents to create children with a set of enhanced traits through genetic engineering. I don't think we will see this soon, but we should discourage the implementation of such practices in our society because of many foreseeable unintended consequences and in order to preserve the richness of diversity we experience today.

Children who are different due to disability are very vulnerable members of our society who deserve to be protected. The area of medical or surgical enhancement of such children is a controversial one, fraught with ethical concerns. Although we can understand the desires of parents who wish to enhance their children's capacities, we remain concerned that by doing so, parents may change the fundamental nature of their child and, in a real sense, affect the world in general by decreasing diversity. Pediatric ethics is often in the business of attempting to create processes that protect vulnerable children from harm. Rarely, we need to protect children from their parents. Parents are, generally, loving and caring people with the best interest of their children at heart. This is certainly true in the context of parents wishing to optimize the capabilities of their children. It may be hard for parents to embrace difference when they are faced with a child who isn't "normal," but most do just that, and become fierce advocates for optimizing their child's future. Attempting to enhance our children may change who they are and who they were destined to become. Some may think we should not attempt to change our children, but rather make the world more accepting of diversity. Parents should not be held responsible for changing the world into which they brought their child. In some circumstances it may be easier to change the fundamental nature of a child to alleviate his or her suffering than it is to change the societal conditions that have produced that suffering. I believe that there are times when loving parents in collaboration with caring physicians are justified in trying to optimize their child's capacities by embarking on an enhancement strategy. At the same time, those of us who care about children who are different can work to decrease stigma and to create a world that is more accepting of diversity.

ADDITIONAL READINGS

Allen DB, Cuttler L. Short stature in childhood—challenges and choices. *N Engl J Med*, 2013; 368: 1220–1228.

Ambler GR, Fairchild J, Wilkinson DJC. Debate: Idiopathic short stature should be treated with growth hormone. *J Paediatr Child Health*, 2012; 49: 165–169.

Goeke J, Kassow D, May D, Kundert D. Parental opinions about facial plastic surgery for individuals with Down Syndrome. *Ment Retard*, 2003; 41: 29–34.

Parens E. Is better always good? The Enhancement Project. *Hastings Center Report*, 1998; 28: S1–S16.

Parens E, Johnston J. Troubled children: diagnosing, treating and attending to context. *Hastings Center Report*, 2011; 41(2): S4–S31.

Robertson JA. Ethics and the future of preimplantation genetic diagnosis. *Ethics, Law Moral Philos Reprod Med*, 2005; 1:97–101.

Solomon A. Dwarfs. In: Far from the tree: parents, children, and the search for identity. New York, NY: Scribner, 2012: 115–167.

Wilfond BS, Miller PS, Korfiatis C, et al. Navigating growth attenuation in children with profound disabilities. *Hastings Center Report*, 2010; 40: 27–40.

CHAPTER 10
Ethical Issues in Research Involving Children

Biomedical and public health research during the 20th century resulted in dramatic changes in maternal and infant mortality, the near eradication of infectious causes of death in childhood, and the conquering of many serious diseases affecting children. There are numerous examples of the successes of science guided by clinical research: the creation of vaccines to eradicate diphtheria, polio, measles, and meningitis; the development of pharmacologic treatment regimens that have changed diabetes, leukemia, and human acquired immunodeficiency disease (HIV/AIDS) from uniformly fatal to chronic diseases; as well as the application of technology and molecular biology to the treatment of profoundly preterm infants.

The potential benefits of research involving children must be balanced with the concern that children require special protection from the risks of research. Unlike adults, young children asked to be participants in research cannot provide informed consent to place themselves at some level of risk with uncertain benefit for the purpose of generating new knowledge that will likely help future children. Although some commentators have questioned whether it is ever ethical to do research involving children, most agree that we should be willing to place children at a reasonable level of risk for the sake of generating important information about childhood

This Chapter has been adapted with permission from Fleischman AR, Collogan L. *Children* In: Emanuel EJ, Grady C, Crouch RA, Lie R, Miller F, Wendler D, eds. *The Oxford Textbook of Clinical Research Ethics*. Oxford University Press; 2008: 446–460.

diseases that could help future children. But if we are going to place children at risk in research studies, we must develop the necessary methods to protect them from undue risk, and to assure that they receive compensating individual benefit whenever possible. Research with animals when possible and research with consenting adults and older children with child assent and parental permission should precede research with young children and infants. But the distinct aspects of childhood diseases, the need to consider the broad range of growth and development, the unique metabolism, and the possibility of unexpected drug toxicities, all require research be conducted with children of all ages to generate scientific and medical advances that enhance the health and well-being of children.

The history of research involving children reveals that the interests of child participants have not always been protected and that researchers have exploited many children. The challenge over the last 30 years has been to create a system of regulation and supervision of research involving children that allows advances in the understanding of the physical, psychological, and social growth and development of children and the pathophysiology and treatment of diseases and disorders that affect children, while protecting the participants from unnecessary and uncompensated risks and discomforts.

HISTORICAL BACKGROUND

Medical research with child subjects is not well documented prior to the development of pediatrics as a medical specialty in the late-19th century. But as early as the 17th century, with the development of modern medicine, physicians began to take an interest in childhood diseases. Entire texts devoted to the treatment of childhood conditions began to appear, and European medical schools began to include instruction in pediatrics. The 17th century also saw the beginning of modern medical research, generally observational in nature, studying disease by recording the clinical course of an illness and attempting to correlate worsening conditions to environmental factors. This type of formal clinical observation led to significant advances in medicine, including the introduction of inoculation for smallpox in the 18th century. A small amount of the smallpox organism was placed subcutaneously to generate protective antibodies in poor English children who were highly susceptible to smallpox. Inoculation became widespread right after members of the British royal family began having the procedure performed on their offspring. In 1796, Edward Jenner conducted his famous smallpox vaccination experiment using cowpox on an 8-year-old patient and other children in his village. Jenner saw his work as highly beneficial, and though he discussed the risks with his subjects and their families, he did not seem troubled by the use of children as research subjects.

Jenner described his work as likely to be valuable to mankind and thus worth the risk to subjects. Jenner's smallpox trials, and other early research projects involving children, were rooted in a sincere desire to benefit society and to help children, a group that historically had been ignored by medical practitioners. The 18th century was a time of dramatic medical advances. It closed with a call for better care for infants and children due to a new appreciation of the serious problem of infant mortality. By the beginning of the 19th century the groundwork had been laid for a new commitment to improved healthcare for children, and for a decrease in infant mortality.

Pediatric medicine formally became a recognized medical specialty in the mid-19th century, and medical societies in the United States and Europe began to form pediatric sections in the 1880s. A growing interest in child health led to the creation of pediatric hospitals that cared for cognitively impaired and disabled children. These institutions, along with orphanages, provided investigators with a ready population of children as subjects of research. There were often outbreaks of various communicable diseases in institutions, and the readily available residents were useful subjects for a growing number of investigations. Within the medical and research communities, there was little objection to research involving institutionalized children and even less concern about informed consent of participants or their parents. Most saw the societal benefits of the research studies as outweighing the potential risks to subjects, particularly for institutionalized subjects whose risk of contracting a communicable disease was very high.

In the 20th century, as with earlier research, many studies in the United States focused on highly communicable diseases such as smallpox, tuberculosis, pertussis, measles, and polio. Other studies examined new diagnostic techniques such as spinal taps and looked at physiology such as stomach emptying time in children to understand differences between children and adults. In contrast to Jenner, pediatric investigators during the early 1900s rarely openly discussed the risks or discomfort to their subjects or mentioned ethical concerns about placing children at risk in research. Investigators rarely justified their work as potentially benefitting the subjects or other children in similar circumstances. Furthermore, as in the previous century, the participants in these studies often were poor or abandoned children provided to researchers by doctors working in orphanages and institutions.

Most medical professionals did not object to the use of children as research subjects, but the antivivisectionist movement, which had long protested the use of animals in medical research, also protested the involvement of children as research subjects. These protests, which began in the late 19th century, included publications devoted to citing research cruelties and pamphlets arguing against research involving children. The protests prompted some lawmakers to propose antivivisection bills that attempted to formally regulate or ban research with live animals, including children.

During World War II, concern over injury and illness among young soldiers created a sharp increase in medical research in the United States. In addition, Nazi doctors in concentration camps conducted numerous medical experiments on human subjects. Many of these experiments had dubious, if any, scientific basis, and experimenters made no attempt to solicit the permission of subjects or explain to them the purpose of the studies. Children were not exempt from experimentation; indeed, some Nazi physicians specifically sought children for studies. Many of these experiments resulted in significant suffering, disability, and death. After the liberation of the concentration camps and the end of the War, many of the physicians and Nazi officials who performed experiments on prisoners in concentration camps were brought to trial at Nuremberg. The American judges at the trial issued the Nuremberg Code, a universal statement intended to ensure the ethical conduct of future research. The Code was a list of 10 governing principles to guide medical experimentation with human subjects. In addition to mandating sound scientific experimental methods, the Code stipulated that the "voluntary consent of the human subject is absolutely essential" and this consent is only valid if the person giving it has the legal capacity to do so. This requirement effectively prohibited any research with children or any other incapacitated individuals, such as those with mental illness or cognitive impairment that limited the capacity to consent. American scientists and clinicians viewed Nazi doctors and the atrocities of the Holocaust as removed from the realities of medicine and experimentation in the United States. The Nuremburg Code was generally ignored in the United States and research with children continued without any real attempts at regulation until the 1970s.

Given the largely indifferent response to the Nuremberg Code in general, and its specific prohibition of research involving children, in the early 1960s, the World Medical Association set about to create a universal set of professional guidelines to aid investigators in conducting ethically sound clinical research. These guidelines were to be created by professionals for professionals and would help to standardize the practices of clinical investigation throughout the developed world. The document was called the Declaration of Helsinki. It created a clear distinction between what was called therapeutic research—research with patients within medical care—and nontherapeutic research— research performed on healthy subjects to gain new knowledge. The final version of the Declaration that was adopted in 1964, allowed both therapeutic and nontherapeutic research to be performed using children, provided consent was obtained from a legal representative of the subject, and assent was obtained from the child when appropriate.

There was growing awareness among professionals, government agencies, and some members of the public that formal research oversight was needed. In 1962, it was discovered that the widespread use of an anti-emetic, thalidomide, recommended for morning sickness in pregnant women, but never tested or approved in the United States, caused severe birth defects. The ensuing scandal caused the Food and Drug Administration to mandate that all new drugs be tested in standardized trials, using formal-consent procedures. In 1963, the director of the National Institutes of Health (NIH) created a committee to review investigations funded under the auspices of the NIH to study problems of consent and unethical practices in clinical research. This committee developed several proposals for consideration by the Public Health Service that resulted, in 1966, in a memorandum from the U.S. Surgeon General to all institutions receiving federal research funds. The memorandum stated that no grants would be funded by the Public Health Service for research involving human beings unless the grantee institution provided prior review by an institutional committee to assure an independent determination that the risks and potential benefits of the investigation, and the methods used to secure informed consent, are appropriate, and that the rights and welfare of the individuals involved will be respected.

Research involving children continued, but two studies exposed in the early 1970s made the public aware of questionable research practices and triggered the creation of government research regulations. The first was a series of studies on the transmission of hepatitis in institutionalized children at the Willowbrook State School, a large hospital for mentally disabled children in Staten Island, New York. Hepatitis was endemic at Willowbrook, and investigators were working to find a way to prevent its spread. This research program was criticized when published studies revealed that healthy children newly admitted to the institution were deliberately infected with hepatitis virus in order to study the spread of the disease and to set the basis for the development of a vaccine for prevention. Investigators defended the work, arguing that exposing children to hepatitis while following a protocol in a special research unit entailed less risk than normal institutional exposure. Although permission for the children to participate was obtained from the parents, critics argued that the consent process was coercive and that the research was clearly exploitation of this institutionalized population.

The second important event was a report in the *New York Times* on the Tuskegee Syphilis Study. This U.S. Public Health Service study was first funded in 1932 as a natural history study of the progression of syphilis in 400 black men in Alabama. Although the Tuskegee study did not include children, it focused attention on the potential for vulnerable populations to be exploited in the context of research. The study was not a secret in the medical community; over the years, it had been reviewed and re-funded by the Public Health Service and several papers were published with results and observations. The men in the study continued to be followed without treatment, even after antibiotics had been found to effectively treat the disease. However, in 1972, when the *New York Times* published an expose documenting the study, there was a public outcry that led to a series of investigations.

In the 1970s, there was a vigorous debate among healthcare providers, researchers, and ethicists about the morality of involving children as participants in research. Paul Ramsey, a Protestant theologian, wrote that research that involved children was only justified if it furthered the medical interests of the individual child subject, and, thus, children should never be involved in research without the potential for direct benefit. In contrast, Richard McCormick, a Catholic theologian, argued that research with children was necessary to improve the health and well-being of all children, and that parental consent was sufficient to protect the interests of individual children exposed to research risks.

McCormick argued further that individuals, even infants, ought to value human life and the health of others, and if they were able to make informed decisions, children would most likely choose to participate in experiments that might contribute to knowledge, as long as the personal risks were not too great. Thus, he maintained that parents and guardians, in the interest of serving what would be the choices of their children, should be able to consent to the participation of their children in research. Many commentators, agreeing with McCormick, argued that enrolling a child in a research study enhanced moral development by doing good for others, just like the common practice of asking a child to contribute a part of his or her allowance to charity each week.

Ramsey vehemently disagreed with McCormick's arguments and maintained that to enroll children in research because they "ought" to help others was to impose adult morality on a population that lacked the capacity to make such decisions. He maintained that being subjects in research could not contribute to the moral growth of children because their participation was unconscious and unwilled. He argued further that any nontherapeutic research participation by persons unable to provide consent, no matter how small the potential risk, was ethically unacceptable. The resolution of this debate required the development of a national consensus, which occurred through the creation of the first national bioethics commission.

THE NATIONAL COMMISSION FOR THE PROTECTION OF SUBJECTS OF RESEARCH

In 1974, Congress passed legislation to create the National Commission for the Protection of Subjects of Biomedical and Behavioral Research, charged with making recommendations about how research should be regulated in the United States. The dilemma of involving children and other vulnerable groups in research was among the most pressing concerns of the Commission. The Commission chose to clarify the basic principles of research ethics in a document called the Belmont Report, published in 1978. Among many important contributions, this report laid out a broad justification of research involving children. The Commission argued that: "Effective ways of treating childhood diseases and fostering healthy development are benefits that serve to justify research involving children—even when individual research subjects are not beneficiaries." The Report went on to explicitly mention a second justification for research involving children: "Research also makes it possible to avoid the harm that may result from the application of previously accepted routine practices that on closer investigation turn out to be dangerous."

Although the Report supported research involving children, it notes that those who are unable to make decisions for themselves are potentially vulnerable and in need of protection from undue influence and coercion. The Commission developed a set of ethical principles that would govern research; perhaps the most important was the principle of respect for persons. This principle incorporates two ethical convictions: first, those individuals with the capacity to make decisions should be treated as autonomous agents able to give permission or to refuse participation in research studies; and second, persons with diminished autonomy are entitled to protection. Children, unable to consent for their own participation in research, require protection. Invoking the authority of parents as surrogate decision-makers is seen as only one aspect of that protection. Careful scrutiny of the level of risk to which a child might be exposed in the research context, and minimizing risks in research whenever possible, were two additional protective approaches outlined in the Report.

In 1977, the National Commission released "Research Involving Children," a report specifically examining the ethical aspects of research with children as subjects.

The Commission noted that the most pressing concern about children as research subjects is their "reduced autonomy" and "incompetency to give informed consent," leaving them vulnerable and unable to protect themselves against unscrupulous research practices. They argued that supporting research involving children is based on the fact that, in numerous instances, there is no suitable alternative population of research subjects; prohibiting research involving children would impede innovative efforts to develop new treatments for diseases that affect children, decrease knowledge of the antecedents of adult disease, and result in the introduction of practices in the treatment of childhood diseases without the benefit of research or evaluation.

The report defines children as "persons who have not attained the legal age of consent to care as determined under the applicable law of the jurisdiction in which the research will be conducted." Such a definition recognizes the local implementation of federal regulations and implies that the recommendations made in the report would vary depending on local and state laws. The definition also highlights that the ability to consent that distinguishes children from adults is not dependent solely on chronologic age.

The Commission directly addresses Ramsey's argument against allowing research involving children that has no therapeutic intent, and rejects his views as overly restrictive and unnecessary to protect the rights and interests of children. The report does, however, recommend specific limitations of permissible research with children, requiring a local Institutional review board (IRB) to determine that:

1. The research is scientifically sound and significant.
2. Where appropriate, studies have been conducted first on animals and adult humans, then on older children, prior to involving infants.
3. Risks are minimized by using the safest procedures consistent with sound research design, and by combining research with standard procedures performed for diagnostic or treatment purposes whenever feasible.

4. Adequate provisions are made to protect the privacy of children and their parents and to maintain confidentiality of the data.
5. Subjects will be selected in an equitable manner.
6. The conditions of all applicable subsequent recommendations are met.

Additional recommendations include discussions of permissible levels of risk, the balancing of risks and potential benefits, the role of parental permission and child assent, and the involvement of children in research who are institutionalized or wards of the state.

U.S. FEDERAL REGULATIONS REGARDING RESEARCH WITH CHILDREN

In 1981, based on the recommendations of the National Commission, Congress adopted the Department of Health and Human Services Policy for Protection of Human Research Subjects. These regulations require institutional review and approval for all research with human participants, as well as voluntary informed consent from subjects or their legally authorized representatives. The regulations apply to all research involving human subjects under the purview of the DHHS and describe in detail the composition, purposes, and procedures for IRBs. In 1983, subpart D of the regulations, Additional Protections for Children Involved as Subjects in Research, was promulgated. The regulations in subpart D have also been adopted with a few exceptions by the Food and Drug Administration for application to clinical drug trials. The National Commission report, Research Involving Children, had a significant impact on creation of this part of the regulations. Much like the National Commission Report, subpart D defines children as "persons who have not attained the legal age for consent to treatments or procedures involved in the research, under the applicable law of the jurisdiction in which the research will be conducted." This definition has significance particularly for adolescents, who, in most jurisdictions, may consent for clinical care and treatment for sexually transmitted diseases, pregnancy and its prevention, and mental health services. Although somewhat controversial and not universally used, IRBs may consider research on these issues that involve adolescents to be reviewed as if the subjects were not children but rather autonomous adults who may consent for participation in research without parental involvement.

The regulations create four categories of permissible research involving children based on the level of risk. In adults, permissibility of research is determined primarily by the participant's ability to understand the risks of the study and to have the capacity to consent; whereas in children, the pediatric regulations limit permissible research based on the degree of risk. In addition, the informed consent of the parent or guardian is required for children. Parents are not allowed to give permission to as wide a range of studies as is permissible for autonomous adult subjects. The first category of permissible research is research deemed to have a risk level of "no greater than minimal," regardless of whether or not there is the prospect of direct benefit to the child. Second, research that holds out the "prospect of direct benefit" to individual subjects is permitted as long as the risks are minimized and justified by the level of compensating benefit. Third, research is permitted if it involves greater-than-minimal risk and no prospect of direct benefit to individual subjects, but only if the level of risk is merely a "minor increase over minimal;" the intervention or procedure presents experiences to subjects that are commensurate with actual or expected medical, dental, psychological, social, or educational situations; and the research is likely to yield generalizable information of vital importance about the subjects' disorder or condition. Fourth, research that is not otherwise approvable under the first three categories but presents an opportunity to understand, prevent, or alleviate a serious problem affecting the health or welfare of children may be permitted by the Secretary of Health and Human Services after expert consultation and opportunity for public review. This regulatory framework imposes a significant limit on the discretion of investigators and parents to permit the participation of children in research that entails more than minimal risk but at the same time does allow much research of importance to the health and well-being of children. Each of these categories requires interpretation of various terms and requirements. Figure 10.1 depicts an algorithm that may be useful in applying the regulations and understanding the components of each category.

I have had the opportunity on two Department of Health and Human Services (DHHS) federal advisory committees and as an expert advisor to an Institute of Medicine (IOM) report committee, to review this four-tiered approach to permissible research in children based on level of risk and benefit. I believe this algorithm is thoughtful and reasonable as a way to balance the need for pediatric research against the need to protect the interests of children. Unfortunately, local IRBs have often misinterpreted the flexibility built into these categories of permissible research and have created undue barriers to well-intentioned researchers who seek to examine important scientific questions.

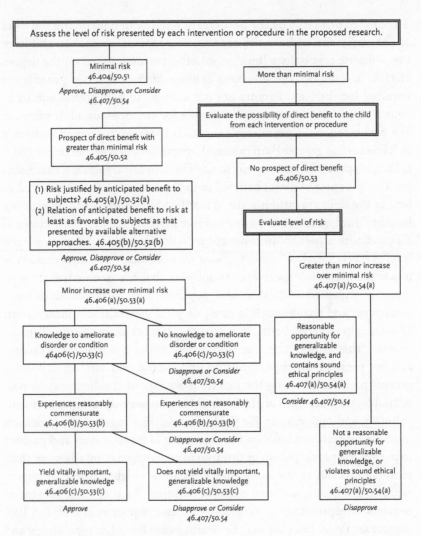

Figure 10.1: Nelson Algorithm for making assessments of research protocols as required by 45 CFR 46.404-407 and 21 CFR 50.51-54.

Research Not Involving Greater Than Minimal Risk

Minimal risk is defined in the regulations in this way: "that the probability and magnitude of harm or discomfort anticipated in the research are not greater in and of themselves than those ordinarily encountered in daily life or during the performance of routine physical or psychological examinations or tests." This definition has been controversial and open to differing interpretations since its adoption over 30 years ago. A 1981 study of pediatric researchers and department chairs, revealed broad disagreement on the level of risk represented by common procedures performed in pediatric practice. More recently, a survey of chairs of IRBs confirmed continued misunderstanding and confusion about this fundamental definition, revealing wide variation of opinion about the risk level associated with such common research procedures as confidential surveys and simple blood draws. Several commentators have criticized the definition of minimal risk for its use of comparisons to the risks encountered in daily life. Clearly, there is a wide range of socially acceptable but risky behaviors that normal, healthy children encounter in their daily lives. These include traveling in cars and buses, bicycle and horseback riding, and playing sports. But few researchers or IRBs have been confused by the intention of the regulations, even if the words allow for misinterpretation: for a procedure to be considered minimal risk, it must have an exceedingly low likelihood of significant or sustained discomfort, irreversible harm, or substantial embarrassment.

Several commentators and a report from the IOM have attempted to clarify the definition of minimal risk. These reports concur that minimal risk should be an objective standard, related neither to the level of illness of the child nor the child's social circumstances. Risks should include all harms, discomforts, indignities, embarrassments, and potential breaches of privacy and confidentiality associated with the research; and minimal risk should be that level of risk associated with the daily activities of a normal, healthy, average child. Indexing the definition of minimal risk to the lives of healthy, average children prevents those higher risks that are routinely experienced by sick children or children exposed to greater risks because of social circumstances, from being considered minimal.

This definition does, however, allow the concept of minimal risk to take into account the changing risks normally experienced by children of different ages. The daily risks encountered in the life of an infant or toddler who is rarely, if ever, left unattended by an adult, differ dramatically from the risks encountered by an adolescent who attends school, drives a car, plays sports, and engages in many independent activities. Research that might be considered to pose greater than minimal risk for a young child (e.g. observation of street-crossing behavior) might be consistent with the risks ordinarily encountered in the daily lives of an older child and thus be considered minimal risk for that population.

The regulatory definition of minimal risk also permits consideration of those experiences encountered by normal, healthy, average children in routine physical and psychological examinations such as those consistent with routine visits to the doctor or dentist or routine psychological testing and observations in school. This allows research procedures such as a simple blood draw, noninvasive urine collection, questionnaires, and interviews with healthy children, as well as magnetic resonance imaging without sedation, to be permissible as minimal risk. When procedures performed once are deemed to be consistent with the definition of minimal risk, the same procedure performed serially or repetitively over a short period may no longer constitute minimal risk because of increased discomfort and the fact that repeated procedures are not consistent with routine visits to the doctor's office.

The definition of minimal risk need not be interpreted literally as only those risks encountered in the actual daily lives of children or their visits to a doctor's office, but may include risks thought to be "equivalent" to those routinely encountered in the daily lives and experiences of normal, healthy, average children. The interpretation of equivalency is left to individual IRBs.

Research Involving Greater Than Minimal Risk but Presenting the Prospect of Direct Benefit to the Individual Subjects

IRBs may approve research that entails more than minimal risk to a child if the intervention or procedure holds out the prospect of direct benefit for the individual subject, and the risk is justified by the anticipated benefit. Most clinical trials fall under this category of research. Many such trials carry a substantial level of risk for the subjects, but the anticipated benefits of treatment of the serious disease against which the research is targeted may warrant the potential risks. This is the crucial balancing required of IRBs. When determining whether a research proposal offers the prospect of direct benefit to individual research subjects, IRBs should ascertain that the benefits to be accrued are derived from the research itself and not the collateral benefits often associated with participation in research. Furthermore, provision of standard clinical care otherwise not available to subjects or monetary compensation for participation in the research should never be considered as a benefit that warrants exposing the subjects to considerable risks.

When assessing the risks imposed by research participation, it is very important to distinguish between those risks associated solely with participation in the research project and those risks inherent in the standard diagnostic approaches and treatments of the disease being studied. To define the incremental risks of the research itself and to determine whether the risks of research participation are reasonable in relation to anticipated benefits, IRBs should do a "component analysis." Through component analysis, the IRB examines each procedure and intervention to determine the therapeutic intent, level of risk, and whether the risks have been sufficiently minimized. Each procedure in a study, if it is not part of standard treatment but presents greater than minimal risk, should be evaluated independently to assure that there is a compensating prospect of direct benefit to the participant from that procedure. If a specific risky procedure (e.g. bone marrow aspirate, spinal tap, imaging with sedation) has no potential to benefit the participant, is only performed to collect data that is solely for research purposes, the IRB may not approve that portion of the research within the category of "prospect of direct benefit."

Research Involving Greater-Than-Minimal Risk and No Prospect of Direct Benefit to Individual Subjects, but Likely to Yield Generalizable Knowledge About the Subject's Disorder or Condition

Research that involves greater-than-minimal risk to children with no prospect of direct benefit is permissible under certain conditions. The research must involve risk that is only a "minor increase over minimal risk," the intervention or procedure must present experiences to the children that are reasonably commensurate with those inherent in their actual or expected medical, dental, psychological, social, or educational situations, and the research must be likely to yield generalizable knowledge about the subjects' disorder or condition that is of vital importance for the understanding or amelioration of that disorder or condition.

The concept of a "minor increase over minimal risk" is contingent on the definition of minimal risk. Minor increase over minimal risk should be interpreted as a very small increment over that level of risk experienced by normal, healthy, average children in their daily lives and experiences. It is not intended that a minor increase over minimal should be defined as the level of risk generally experienced by children who are ill or in socially compromised circumstances. It is the role of the investigator to make the case, and the role of the IRB to review the evidence that research proposed under this category meets the standard of providing generalizable information of "vital importance," and that the procedures are reasonably commensurate with the prior or expected experiences of the subjects.

The definition of "disorder or condition" also requires interpretation. A condition affecting children should be understood more broadly than a specific disease or diagnostic category. It refers to a specific set of physical, psychological, neurodevelopmental, or social characteristics that have been shown to affect children's health and well being, or to increase their risk of developing a health problem in the future. This definition of condition can include a genetic or familial predisposition to future illness, or even a social circumstance that has been linked to a potential deficit in future health and well-being. It is the responsibility of the investigator to substantiate that there is an established body of scientific evidence or clinical knowledge that supports that association.

Research Not Otherwise Approvable That Presents an Opportunity to Understand, Prevent, or Alleviate a Serious Problem Affecting the Health and Welfare of Children

Federal regulations are intended to limit research that involves significant risks to subjects without compensating benefits. However, the regulations do create a process for review of credible research that may not be approved at the local level under the first three categories but that has the potential to significantly affect child health and welfare. An IRB may determine that, although a proposed study may not be approved under the minimal-risk, prospect-of-direct-benefit, or minor-increase-over-minimal-risk categories, the research has a reasonable opportunity to further the understanding, prevention, or alleviation of a serious problem affecting the health or welfare of children. In these rare cases, the IRB may send the proposal to the Office for Human Research Protection, DHHS, or to the Food and Drug Administration, requesting review and approval by the Secretary of Health and Human Services. The Secretary must consult with a panel of experts and assure public review and comment before determining if the research should be permitted to proceed. This procedure had been used rarely in the past, but in recent years a more efficient review process has been developed, which has resulted in somewhat more frequent usage.

Minimizing Risk

It is the duty of all research investigators and the IRB to ensure that risks are minimized in research. This is particularly relevant to research involving children. Even in research studies that involve minimal risk, or a minor increase over minimal risk, every attempt should be made to minimize risk. Research procedures should be integrated with clinical care and diagnostic procedures whenever feasible in order to avoid duplication of uncomfortable procedures and interventions. Procedures should be performed only by professionals who are skilled with children. Protocols should include specific rules that set limits on the number of unsuccessful attempts at a procedure or the length of time for completion of a questionnaire. Appropriate methods should be used to orient children to the research environment and to decrease anxiety and discomfort whenever possible.

In determining whether a proposed procedure has adequately minimized risks, the IRB should take into consideration the context in which the research will be performed. The research environment, the population under study, the experience of the investigator, and the skill of the professionals, all influence the level of risk of each proposed procedure. Specific groups of children may experience certain procedures with greater anxiety, or discomfort as compared to other groups. Children who are cognitively impaired, emotionally disturbed, or mentally ill are likely to experience simple procedures such as a blood draw as deeply disconcerting. A blood test with such children might be considered a greater-than-minimal-risk procedure, unless efforts are made to ameliorate their distress.

Parental (or Guardian) Permission and Child Assent

Informed consent remains the cornerstone of protection of human subjects, even in research involving children. However, since children are generally not capable of providing informed consent, the process of obtaining consent for children is best viewed as parental or guardian permission, with the child's assent when appropriate. The term *parental permission* is used because, in research as in clinical care, parents consenting for children do not have the same rights as capacitated adults consenting for themselves. An IRB may determine that permission of one parent is sufficient for research involving either minimal risk research or research that provides the prospect of direct benefit to the individual child. However, the permission of both parents is required when research involves a minor increase over minimal risk and no prospect of direct benefit, or when the research required the approval of the secretary of DHHS. The requirement for both parents' consent may be altered if one parent is deceased, unknown, incompetent, or not readily available, or when only one parent has legal responsibility for the care and custody of the child.

Parental permission is required for all research involving children, except in a few specific circumstances. Waiver of parental permission may be approved in circumstances similar to the waiver of informed consent for adult participants in research. These circumstances include research conducted by local governments to evaluate public benefit or service programs, or research that involves no more than minimal risk that could not practicably be carried out without the waiver. In this circumstance, the waiver must not adversely affect the rights and welfare of the subjects, and whenever, appropriate, the subjects or their parents should be provided with additional pertinent information after participation. Food and Drug Administration regulations do not allow the waiver of parental permission in drug or device research trials regardless of the level of risk.

There are additional circumstances that may permit waiver of parental permission. Although it is generally beneficial to include parents in decisions about the care of their children, there are situations in which involving parents in the medical care of their child may be detrimental to the child's best interest. In virtually every state, there are laws to permit medical treatment for specific conditions in adolescents (such as sexually transmitted disease, mental illness, and pregnancy) with the consent of the young person and without informing the parents. Waiving parental involvement in consent can be appropriate in the research context as well. Federal regulations permit IRBs to forego parental involvement in research when "parental or guardian permission is not a reasonable requirement to protect the subjects." This could permit waiver of parental permission in cases involving child abuse or neglect or when revealing certain behaviors or illnesses to their parents might hurt adolescents. In each case, the IRB must assure that the investigator will both assess the capacity of adolescents to understand the research and their own rights as subjects, and has created appropriate procedural safeguards (such as the availability of a counselor independent of the research) to protect the interests of the adolescent participants.

In addition to obtaining parental permission, researchers working with children must solicit the child's assent when appropriate. Assent is defined as "a child's affirmative agreement to participate in research." Institutional review boards must take into account the age, maturity, and psychological state of the children involved in the research when determining whether assent will be required. Institutional review board practices vary widely in interpreting the regulations concerning assent. If a child does not provide affirmative agreement or fails to respond, assent cannot be assumed. Not all children, especially those who are very young, are able to provide assent. Institutional review boards may determine that all children in a particular protocol must assent to participate, or that children above a certain age (e.g. six or seven) must assent, or that each child must be assessed individually for the capacity to provide assent. Assent is not required if the research intervention or procedure involved in the research holds out the prospect of direct benefit that is important to the health or well-being of the participants, and is available only in the context of the research. Assent from children may be waived by IRBs, just as informed consent may be waived for adults.

The assent process must be age and developmentally appropriate, and should be an empowering and affirming experience for the child. Assent should not directly parallel the informed consent process for adults. Assent is not "consent-lite," and there is no need to duplicate all the essential elements required in adult informed consent during the assent process. Obtaining assent includes making the child aware of his medical condition (when appropriate), informing him or her about what to expect from the research study, assessing his or her ability to understand the situation, and asking him or her whether or not he or she is willing to take part in the research. Assent need not include a written form or a signature. The assent process should describe, from the perspective of the child, what will happen and what discomforts might be involved in the research. Of course, as the age of the child participants increases, assent information should become more substantive and specific, and begin to resemble an adult informed consent.

I believe that some researchers and some IRBs have interpreted the regulations to require assent in all research involving children above 6 years of age. This practice can create a serious problem in therapeutic studies that have the potential of direct benefit for the subjects. If parents would like their children to participate, but children are asked to assent and refuse, investigators can either respect that refusal and not enroll the child regardless of parental preference, or ignore the refusal and disrespect the child's preference. Agreeing to the child's refusal to participate can result in not being able to enroll a sufficient number of subjects in certain clinical trials for treatment of rare disorders. In the case of research that provides the prospect of direct benefit that is available only in the context of the research, child assent is not a requirement. In such cases, children should still be informed about the research, but not asked for their assent if lack of affirmative agreement to participate will not be respected. It is disrespectful of children to ignore their preferences after they have been solicited. This can result in lack of trust in the physician, the child's parents, and the research enterprise.

Wards

The final section of subpart D concerns research with children who are wards. There is no definition of "wards" in the regulations but it is taken to mean children who do not have a parent or legal guardian from whom permission for enrollment in the research may be obtained. Such children could be institutionalized or in foster care, and the state or local social-service agencies are legally responsible for them. The regulations permit wards to be enrolled in research that involves no greater than minimal risk or that has the prospect of direct benefit, without additional protections. However, wards may be enrolled in research that involves a minor increase over minimal risk with no prospect of direct benefit or in research approved by the Secretary DHHS, only if the research is related to the subjects' status as wards, or is to be "conducted in schools, camps, hospitals, institutions, or similar settings in which the majority of children involved as subjects are not wards." Such research also requires the appointment of an advocate to act in the child's best interest during the child's participation in the research. The advocate may not be associated with the research, the investigators, or the institution legally responsible for the child. This section both permits wards to be enrolled in research that might be in their interests, and also protects the group who had been historically exploited by research investigators.

INCENTIVES, COMPENSATION, PAYMENT

Compensation of pediatric research subjects and their families has long been a controversial issue. Federal regulations on the protection of human subjects of research do not explicitly mention compensation and payments related to participation in research studies. However, investigators often feel that financial inducements are essential to enhance recruitment and retention, particularly in studies that provide no direct benefit to participants. Some commentators believe that children should never be paid for research participation because payment might be an undue inducement and affect the voluntariness of their participation. Similarly they argue that parents ought not to be paid to enroll their children in research, for fear that children will be used as commodities and placed at undue risk for the sake of parental financial gain.

The basic concern is balancing the need to make participation in studies attractive to children and their parents, particularly when there is no prospect of direct individual benefit, with the desire to protect children from being enrolled in potentially risky studies because of an undue financial inducement. Compensation of participants and their parents may be considered in two general categories: reimbursement of any incremental costs of participation in the research and inducements to participate.

It seems unfair to ask parents and children to bear additional costs that result from participation in research. Reimbursement for expenses directly related to research participation such as travel, parking, meals, and child care seem warranted and can be calculated based on real out-of-pocket costs to the families or based on a reasonable estimate of average costs. Payment of lost wages for an older child or a parent as a result of participation in the research is often considered a reasonable reimbursement since lost wages will undoubtedly be a substantial disincentive to participation. However, the level of reimbursement should not exceed the actual lost income due to participation.

There are three types of possible inducements to participate: compensation for time spent in participation, enticements for recruitment and retention, and gifts of appreciation at the completion of the study. I believe that each of these types of inducements can be ethically justified if reasonable. It is generally agreed that individuals who participate in research with the major motivation of benefiting others and no prospect of direct benefit to themselves may receive some additional incentive for participation. A small token gift to the child as a thank you for participation in research is common in such situations. Because larger gifts to the parent or child might unduly influence participation, it is generally acceptable to vary the value of the gift based on the length of time required by the research, but not based on the level of risk. A modest incentive for each activity in a study is a common practice but may become an undue inducement if the cumulative amount is excessive and able to influence voluntary participation.

The Office for Human Research Protection (DHHS) Guidebook discusses IRB responsibilities in assuring that consent is truly voluntary, uncoerced, and not unduly influenced by external factors, including payment. In some of its review and criticism of institutional compliance with federal regulations, the Office for Human Research Protection (OHRP) has opined that enrollment procedures do not adequately address the possibility of undue influences, and that IRBs should recognize the provision of free care as a potential undue influence on voluntary participation in research. IRBs need to be held accountable for this aspect of their review, but should permit some inducements for recruitment and retention and some reasonable gifts of appreciation. In attempts to protect the interests of children we should not demean them by disrespecting their time commitments and not appropriately thanking them for their participation.

The Food and Drug Administration offers specific guidelines for review of compensation in the case of clinical drug trials. The FDA requires that IRBs review and approve all amounts, methods, and timing of payments to subjects to assure that there is no coercion or undue influence on participation. In addition, payment should accrue as the study progresses and not be contingent on the subject completing the entire study. However, a reasonable bonus for the completion of the study is acceptable as long as the IRB determines that the amount is not so large as to unduly induce subjects to stay in the study when they would otherwise have withdrawn. A report from the American Academy of Pediatrics suggests that if remuneration is to be given directly to a child participating in a research study, it is best if it is not discussed until after the study so as not to affect voluntary participation. The report also recommends that reimbursement for medical costs associated with treatment under a research protocol be permitted in certain circumstances. This practice may be an undue influence on participation, but in some special circumstances may be warranted. The potential of this type of compensation to unduly influence poor and uninsured families to be part of research studies must be carefully considered by the IRB in its deliberations.

Compensation for Injury

Federal regulations require that, for research involving more than minimal risk, informed consent must include a statement concerning whether any compensation or medical treatment will be available if injury occurs as part of the research. No federal law or regulation requires or provides compensation for research-related injury. Most research involving children does not offer compensation for non-negligent injury that might occur during a research study. Although this issue is not unique to child participants in research, it seems especially unfair that children who are enrolled in research without their autonomous consent and who might be subject to long-term disability due to the research, without any compensation from the investigators or sponsors. An IOM report concerning research that involves children recommends that research organizations and sponsors pay the medical and rehabilitation costs for children injured as a direct result of research participation, without regard to fault. I agree with this recommendation. This practice is unlikely to become commonplace unless there is a federal law that requires it, and the development of a no-fault insurance pool for such purposes.

SPECIAL POPULATIONS

Adolescents

Although federal regulations regarding research with children apply to all individuals under the legal age of consent to medical treatment for the procedures involved in the research, there has been growing concern about how these protections ought to pertain to adolescents. Adolescents are individuals between 10 and 18 years of age, and their constant state of physiological and psychological development sets them apart from younger children and adults. This population has a number of unique health-related needs and behavioral risks that deserve the attention of the research community. In addition, many adolescents are unwilling to take part in research if disclosing their illness, condition, or behaviors to their parents or guardians is required. As a result, studies that involve substance abuse, mental health, sexual activity, and pregnancy often lack sufficient adolescent participation, and study results may not be applicable to this population.

Some adolescents do not require the involvement of parents in decision-making about their participation in research. Some teens are legally emancipated, below the legal age of majority but working, living outside the home, and sufficiently independent to be treated like adults. Waiver of parental permission for other teens is also permitted. The definition of *children* in the federal regulations includes those not legally allowed to consent to treatment involved in the research, so an IRB could waive parental involvement in providing permission and accept the consent of an adolescent for enrollment in research studies related to certain specific medical areas such as sexually transmitted diseases, mental illness, substance abuse, pregnancy, and birth control. Institutional review boards may also consider waiving parental involvement in decision-making when informing parents about the health-related issues under study may jeopardize the child.

The IOM report on research involving children recommends that IRBs consider waivers of parental permission in informed consent for research when: (a) the research is important to the health and well-being of adolescents and cannot be reasonably or practically carried out without the waiver or (b) the research involves treatments or procedures that state laws permit adolescents to receive without parental permission. In addition, the investigator should be required to present evidence that the adolescents are capable of understanding the research and their rights as research participants, and the research protocol includes appropriate safeguards to protect the interests of the adolescent consistent with the risk presented by the research. This approach, consistent with federal regulations, has received widespread support.

Neonates

Neonates and young infants are subject to the federal regulations in subpart D that specifically addresses the interests of all children. In addition to subpart D, there is another part of the federal regulations, subpart B that is concerned with pregnant women, fetuses, and neonates. In November of 2001, a revised section of subpart B was published concerning nonviable neonates or neonates of uncertain viability involved in research. These additional regulations have the potential to be confusing because of some overlap with subpart D. The primary purpose of subpart B is to regulate research involving pregnant women and fetuses and, in addition, describes regulations pertinent to nonviable fetuses after delivery.

Definitions in subpart B create some additional challenges for pediatric research. A nonviable neonate is defined in the regulations as "a neonate after delivery that, although living, is not viable." Viable is defined as "being able, after delivery, to survive (given the benefit of available medical therapy) to the point of independently maintaining heartbeat and respiration." The difficulty for pediatric investigators and IRBs is the fact that much neonatal research involves extremely premature neonates, at gestational ages of 22–26 weeks, who are considered potentially viable but uncertain in terms of whether they will survive over the long term. The regulations in subpart D have adequately protected the interests of these babies who participate in research, but now provisions of subpart B must also be applied to this population.

For research involving neonates of uncertain viability, subpart B requires that the research hold out the prospect of enhancing the probability of survival of the neonate to the point of viability or that the purpose of the research is the development of important biomedical knowledge that cannot be obtained by other means. In addition, subpart B requires that there will be no added risk to the neonate resulting from the research. This provision of subpart B could be interpreted to be in direct conflict with the minimal risk and minor increase over minimal risk standards discussed in subpart D. Thus, for research that does not offer the prospect of direct benefit to the participants, IRBs must interpret the "no added risk" standard of subpart B rather than the "minimal risk" standard of subpart D when evaluating research that involves neonates of uncertain viability.

In general, I think IRBs should ignore subpart B when reviewing neonatal research and use this subpart only when reviewing research related to pregnancy, fetal development, and previable liveborn neonates.

Economically or Educationally Disadvantaged Children

Many of the most serious illnesses and conditions affecting children are disproportionately represented in those who are economically and educationally disadvantaged. Much important research is focused on preventing and ameliorating these conditions. Children who are economically disadvantaged have multiple vulnerabilities including living in poor neighborhoods, substandard housing, poor access to healthcare, and low-quality schools. Their families are more likely to be immigrants and members of minority groups who experience racism and discrimination. These factors make research with disadvantaged children fraught with potential ethical problems. The relative lack of social, economic, and political power of low-income families can affect the voluntary nature of informed consent, and the educational disadvantage of such families may affect their understanding of the nature of the research. Economically disadvantaged families are also more likely to suffer from "therapeutic misconception," confusing research studies with clinical care.

One approach might be to exclude socioeconomically vulnerable children from research in order to protect them from the potential for exploitation and harm. I believe this approach might protect some children, but it would also deprive many children from being part of studies that will determine the best ways to enhance all children's well being. Research can be viewed as a burdensome enterprise with substantial risk, but it can also be viewed as an activity that provides potential benefits to individuals and to affected populations. Vulnerable populations should be permitted to participate in research when appropriate but additional scrutiny and procedural safeguards may be required to assure their protection from harm. Fairness requires that all children who are affected by a condition, whether rich or poor, be offered the opportunity to contribute to research. The burdens of the research and the benefits of the findings should be distributed among all those who might benefit. It is most important to consider involving disadvantaged children in studies that have the potential to improve the circumstances in which they live and provide knowledge about the social determinants of their health.

Institutional review boards that review research involving vulnerable poor and minority children must give special scrutiny to these proposals to ensure that the balance of risks to benefits in the research is acceptable, that there is not undue inducement to participation, and that parents are well informed and supported in making truly voluntary choices about the participation of their children.

Victims of Terror and Trauma

Disasters, whether they are unintentional acts of nature or human produced terror, can have profound effects on the victims. Much can be learned from research conducted in the aftermath of disaster to assist affected individuals, and to help develop preventive and responsive interventions for the future. Although research has defined the many ways in which survivors of terror and trauma are affected physically and emotionally, there is less known about the affect of research participation itself on the survivors. Disaster victims are often viewed as exceptionally vulnerable as research participants. The concept of vulnerability in research has been applied to populations who may have characteristics that impair their ability to provide voluntary and uncoerced informed consent, so that they may be more likely to be taken advantage of as participants in research. Disaster victims and their families frequently suffer from significant psychological and emotional distress and may show signs of acute anxiety, depression, post-traumatic stress, and severe grief. These factors combined with the additional stresses of dislocation, social disruption, and financial strain, may make some individuals and parents unable to provide informed consent to participation in research. However, as a class, disaster victims and their families should not be assumed to be impaired and unable to participate knowingly and voluntarily in decision-making concerning research participation.

There are data to support that some potential research participants will have impaired decision-making capacity as a result of their traumatic experience; however, it would be inappropriate to assume that disaster victims and their families are all decisionally impaired and should be precluded from participation in research. Some have argued that there are significant risks involved in participating in research postdisaster because of rekindling memories of the traumatic events. This fear of "retraumatization"—the reactivation or intensification of stress-related symptoms precipitated by triggered memories—may occur in the clinical or research setting. But the stress of retraumatization should not be confused with the stress caused by the actual occurrence of traumatic exposure. In fact, many victims of terror and trauma appreciate the attention paid to them by researchers and may actually benefit from being able to retell their stories.

After the Oklahoma City and New York World Trade Center disasters, I had the opportunity to help create a series of national recommendations concerning how best to deal with protection of research subjects postterror and trauma. These recommendations include the following: (a) the assumption that affected victims and their families have the capacity to provide informed consent for research participation unless they are assessed to be incapacitated; (b) information for potential subjects should make every effort to decrease therapeutic misconception by making clear whether there is therapeutic intent in the research to decrease the possibility of mistaking research for clinical services; and (c) proposals should have explicit plans for training and support of research staff to identify and ameliorate any untoward events to research subjects of participation.

FINAL THOUGHTS

In recent years, several regulatory and legislative initiatives have increased funding for research involving children in the United States and have created incentives to the pharmaceutical industry to study drugs in children. The pediatric research community and many advocates for children have applauded these changes as long overdue programs to enhance the health of children. Others have voiced concern about increasing research in children because they believe the present human-subjects protection system is generally inadequate to protect the interests of participants in research. Children, particularly vulnerable because of their limited capacity for informed consent, are felt to require even more special protections.

Those who criticize the system for protection of children involved in research claim that increased federal funding and incentives to pharmaceutical companies result in healthy children being subjected to undue risks and sick children being enrolled in trials that provide more benefit to the pharmaceutical industry sponsor than to the child participants. They argue that IRBs are not properly evaluating the level of risk in protocols and are approving studies not in the interests of participants. None of the recent initiatives to increase funding for research in children have weakened the federal regulations that govern research that involves children.

There are some aspects of the system to protect child participants in research that would benefit from clarification, as has been suggested in reports from the IOM, but I believe the fundamental structure of the system to protect children as participants in research is sound and appears to be working well.

The quality of IRB reviews of individual protocols varies greatly, and there is general agreement about a need for accreditation of IRBs and better education of its members to increase quality, uniformity, and accountability. There is also the need to develop performance measures to evaluate the entire human subjects review system. Research-ethics consultation has become available to pediatric investigators in a few of the leading academic medical centers across the country. This type of guidance to assist researchers to ensure ethically designed and implemented protocols, as well as high quality consent and assent processes, can be extremely helpful to participants, researchers, and IRBs. Academic medical centers should encourage this practice in order to facilitate research that involves children.

Well-designed and well-executed research that involves children is essential to improve the health of today's children and tomorrow's adults. Investigators, sponsors, IRBs, research institutions, regulators, and government policymakers all play critical roles in facilitating excellence in research and ensuring participants are appropriately protected.

ADDITIONAL READINGS

Collogan LK, Fleischman AR. Adolescent research and parental permission. In: Kodish E., ed., *Ethics and Research with Children*. New York, NY: Oxford University Press; 2005: 77–99.

Collogan LK, Tuma F, Dolan-Sewell R, Borja S, Fleischman AR. Ethical issues pertaining to research in the aftermath of disaster. *J Traum Stress*, 2004; 17: 363–372.

Department of Health and Human Services. Final regulations concerning protection of human subjects, 45CFR46. http://www.hhs.gov/ohrp

Fleischman AR, and Collogan L.: Children. In: Emanuel EJ, Grady C, Crouch RA, Lie R, Miller F, D Wendler D, eds., *The Oxford Textbook of Clinical Research Ethics*. Oxford University Press;, 2008: 446–460. http://www.hhs.gov.fda/humansubjects

Food and Drug Administration. 21CFR 50 and 56

Institute of Medicine. Ethical conduct of research involving children. Washington, DC: The National Academies Press; 2004.

Grodin MA, Alpert JJ. Children as participants in medical research. *Ped Clin N Am*, 1988; 35: 1389–1401.

Lederer SE. Children as guinea pigs: Historical perspective. *Accountabil Res*, 2003; 10: 1–16.

National Commission. *The Belmont Report: Ethical Principles and Guidelines for the Protection of Human Subjects of Research.* Washington DC: U.S. Government Printing Office; 1978.

National Commission, Report and Recommendations: *Research Involving Children.* Washington DC: U.S. Government Printing Office; 1977.

Nuremberg Code: Directives for human experimentation. In: *Trials of War Criminals Before the Nuremberg Military Tribunals Under Control Council Law No. 10 Vol 2.* Washington, DC: U.S. Government Printing Office; 1949.

World Medical Association. *Declaration of Helsinki,* 1964.

INDEX

beneficence
in pediatric ethics, 6–7
pregnancy-related, 43–44
beneficence-based obligations, 58–60
in changing health-risking behaviors
during pregnancy, 58–60
of clinicians to adolescent alone, 164
of clinicians to patients, 147
of clinicians treating adolescents, 159
to fetus, 44, 59–60
to neonates, 44
to pregnant women, 43–44
term delivery–related, 48
biobank(s). *see also* biobanking
described, 101–104
information technology infrastructures associated with, 102
IRBs of, 103, 105
participation in
blanket consent for, 104
by children, 105–106
informed consent for, 103–106
no direct benefits from, 104–105
privacy in, 102
research findings from
revealing *vs.* withholding of,
106–108
biobanking, 101–108. *see also* biobank(s)
critics of, 102–103
ethical issues related to, 102–108
population-based, 102
privacy in, 102
risks of breaches of, 102–103
bioethics, 5–6
defined, 5
described, 5
principles in, 6–8. *see also* principle(s)
bioethics committees
infant
ethical issues in, 69–71. *see also*
infant bioethics committees
bioethics program for infants
at Montefiore Medical Center, 4
birth
giving
ethical issues related to, 41–60. *see*
also giving birth, ethical issues
related to
good
described, 42

birth asphyxia
death related to
window of opportunity
for, 77–79
described, 77
in neonatal intensive care, 77–79
prognosis for recovery
from, 77–78
birth plans
creation of
clinicians' role in, 46–47
blanket consent
for biobank participation, 104
blood
extra
in newborn screening, 98–101
body image
of adolescents, 172
brain damage
irreversible upper
resumption of breathing and, 79
brain dead mother
problems related to maintaining body
in stable physiologic state
to allow fetus to develop to
viability, 57–58
ethical issues related to, 57–58
brain death
in children, 117–120
American Academy of Pediatrics
on, 117–118
case example, 113, 118
concept of, 117
ethical issues related to, 118–120
guidelines for clinical determination of, 117
organ donation and, 119–120
concept of
development of, 117
defined, 117
maternal catastrophe and
ethical issues related to, 55–58
in pregnant woman, 56
breathing
resumption of
irreversible upper brain damage
related to, 79
Brown, L., 18
bulimia
among adolescents, 172–173

cancer
  in children conceived with IVF, 20
  treatment for
    freezing and storing gametes
      for future use in patients
      undergoing, 30–31
"candidate genes," 86–87
Catholic tradition
  assisted reproduction and, 16–17
CDC. *see* Centers for Disease Control
      and Prevention (CDC)
Centers for Disease Control and
      Prevention (CDC)
  on fertility programs, 21–22
Centers for Medicare and Medicaid
      Services (CMS), 153
cesarean section
  elective
    ethical issues related to, 47–48
  postmortem
    newborns born by, 55–56
    threshold of viability and, 51–52
cessation of circulatory function
  irreversibility of, 120–121
  reversibility of, 120–121
chemotherapy
  freezing and storing gametes for future
      use in patients undergoing, 30–31
chickenpox immunization
  refusal of, 136
child. *see also* children
  creating of
    ethical issues in, 12–40. *see also*
      creating child, ethical issues in
  death of
    supporting family after, 131–132
  dying
    care of, 130–131
child abuse
  examination for, 143–144
  reporting suspected, 143–144
    ethical issues related to, 143–144
    hesitancy in, 144
    procedure for, 143–144
Child Abuse Prevention and Treatment
      Act Amendments, 67–69
child assent
  defined, 212
  for research involving children,
      211–213

children. *see also* child
  biobank participation by, 105–106
  born in U.S. annually, 13
  brain death in, 117–120. *see also* brain
      death, in children
  clinicians keeping important
      information from, 129
  critically ill. *see* critically ill children
  defined, 203, 204, 217
  economically or educationally
      disadvantaged
    research involving, 219–220
  end-of-life care participation by
    case example, 113–114, 128, 129
    ethical issues related to, 127–129
  as family's property, 9
  genetic testing and screening in,
      83–112. *see also* genetic testing
      and screening
  gravely ill
    caring for, 113–133. *see also*
      end-of-life care
  moral and legal status of
    in America, 9–10
  mortality data, 114
  parental requests for keeping
      important information from
    myths and misconceptions about,
      128–129
  parental values and behaviors
    criticized by, 2
  as persons, 9
  poverty among, 10
  reasons for having, 2
  research involving
    ethical issues in, 196–233. *see also*
      research involving children
  rights of, 9
  as special, 1–11
Christian Science
  on refusal of medically indicated
      treatments, 134, 141–142
chromosomal disorders
  genetic testing and screening for, 87
Church of Jesus Christ of Latter Day
      Saints
  assisted reproduction and, 17
circulatory death
  organ donation after
    ethical issues related to, 120–122

personal
   basis for, 3
   in decision-making in neonatal
      intensive care, 74
   physician's
      basis for, 3–4
      on whom to serve, 23, 25
   "transfers" of, 153
varicella (chickenpox) immunization
   refusal of, 136
viability
   threshold of. *see* threshold of viability
viable
   defined, 218
"virtually futile in terms of survival," 68

Wakefield, A., 139–140
ward(s)
   described, 214

research on
   ethical issues in, 214
whole genome testing, 86
   American College of Medical Genetics
      on, 109
   case example, 109
   ethical issues related to, 108–111
Willowbrook State School, 200
window of opportunity
   birth asphyxia–related, 77–79
   in neonatal intensive care, 77–79
withholding of medical treatment
   indications for, 68
withholding *vs.* withdrawal of
      treatment
   in end-of-life care, 123–124

Yale University School of Medicine,
      65–66